FUNDAMENTAL NURSING PROCEDURES

Rita Tobler, RN, MSN

Ms. Tobler, author of this book, is an Assistant Professor of Nursing and First Level Coordinator at Northern Kentucky University, Highland Heights. She received her BSN from the University of Dayton (Ohio) and her MSN from the University of California, San Francisco. Ms. Tobler is a member of the National League for Nursing, the American Nurse's Association, and the American Association of University Professors.

Mae E. Timmons, RN, EdD

Ms. Timmons, reviewer of this book, is an Assistant Professor of Nursing at the University of San Francisco School of Nursing. She received her diploma in nursing from St. John's Hospital School of Nursing, Springfield, Missouri, her BSN from St. Louis University School of Nursing, her MN from the University of California, Los Angeles, and her EdD from the University of San Francisco. Ms. Timmons is a member of the National League for Nursing, the California League for Nursing, the American Nurses' Association, California Nurses' Association, and Sigma Theta Tau, Beta Gamma Chapter.

Springhouse Corporation
Springhouse, Pennsylvania

Staff

Executive Director, Editorial
Stanley Loeb

Director of Trade and Textbooks
Minnie B. Rose, RN, BSN, MEd

Art Director
John Hubbard

Clinical Consultant
Maryann Foley, RN, BSN

Editors
David Moreau, Karen Zimmermann

Copy Editor
Mary Hohenhaus Hardy

Designers
Stephanie Peters (associate art director),
Jacalyn Facciolo

Art Production
Robert Perry (manager), Anna Brindisi, Donald
Knauss, Tom Robbins, Robert Wieder

Typography
David Kosten (director), Diane Paluba (manager),
Elizabeth Bergman, Joyce Rossi Biletz, Phyllis
Marron, Robin Rantz, Valerie L. Rosenberger

Manufacturing
Deborah Meiris (manager), T.A. Landis,
Jennifer Suter

Contents

How to Use Springhouse Notes

Today, more than ever, nursing students face enormous time pressures. Nursing education has become more sophisticated, increasing the difficulties students have with studying efficiently and keeping pace.

The need for a comprehensive, well-designed series of study aids is great, which is why we've produced Springhouse Notes...to meet that need. Springhouse Notes provide essential course material in outline form, enabling the nursing student to study more effectively, improve understanding, achieve higher test scores, and get better grades.

Key features appear throughout each book, making the information more accessible and easier to remember.
- **Learning Objectives.** These objectives precede each section in the book to help the student evaluate knowledge before and after study.
- **Key Points.** Highlighted in gray throughout the book, these points provide a way to quickly review critical information. Key points may include:
  - a cardinal sign or symptom of a disorder
  - the most current or popular theory about a topic
  - a distinguishing characteristic of a disorder
  - the most important step of a process
  - a critical assessment component
  - a crucial nursing intervention
  - the most widely used or successful therapy or treatment.
- **Points to Remember.** This information, found at the end of each section, summarizes the section in capsule form.
- **Glossary.** Difficult, frequently used, or sometimes misunderstood terms are defined for the student at the end of each section.

Remember: Springhouse Notes are learning tools designed to *help* you. They are not intended for use as a primary information source. They should never substitute for class attendance, text reading, or classroom note-taking.

This book, *Fundamental Nursing Procedures,* uses the nursing process and basic needs as a framework for discussing nursing procedures. The text addresses such basic client needs as hygiene, safety, mobility, and elimination and outlines the nursing procedures associated with each. Medication administration, I.V. therapy, wound care, heat and cold applications, and oxygenation are also discussed. Essential steps and nursing considerations are listed for each procedure.

Introduction to Nursing

Learning Objectives

After studying this section, the reader should be able to:

- Define nursing.

- Describe the five steps of the nursing process.

- Provide examples of independent, dependent, and inter-dependent nursing actions.

- Discuss Maslow's needs theory.

- Identify the essential components common to all nursing procedures.

I. Introduction to Nursing

A. Overview of nursing

1. Nursing is the art and science of caring for clients
   a. Nurses help clients to attain, maintain, or restore health
   b. Nurses apply expert knowledge and skill to client care
2. The nursing process—a systematic, scientific approach to planning and providing nursing care—consists of five steps:
   a. Assessment
   b. Diagnosis
   c. Planning
   d. Implementation
   e. Evaluation
3. During implementation, the nurse performs actions to meet the client's basic needs and promote healthy physiologic responses
4. Nursing actions (also called nursing orders or nursing interventions) can be independent, dependent, or interdependent
   a. *Independent* nursing actions are planned by a nurse based on knowledge and skills (for example, teaching and counseling); a physician's order is not required
   b. *Dependent* nursing actions are dictated by medical practice and require the direct order of a physician (for example, administering medication)
   c. *Interdependent* nursing actions are performed or planned in collaboration with other health care professionals, such as physical or respiratory therapists (for example, performing postural drainage)
5. Some nursing actions require specific nursing care procedures to meet client needs
   a. Nurses must have basic knowledge of these procedures to maintain client safety
   b. Nurses must be skilled in performing basic actions to maintain client comfort and attain the desired outcome of the procedure

B. Basic human needs

1. General information
   a. A need is something necessary for an individual's life or well-being, and meeting needs is essential to the physiologic and emotional health of humans
   b. Unmet needs can place a client at risk for illness, whereas fulfilling needs helps maintain or restore health
   c. Abraham Maslow developed a needs theory that arranges basic human needs in order of their importance to survival
   d. Maslow's needs theory (or an adaptation, such as Kalish's) is commonly used as a component of a nursing conceptual framework

2. Maslow's hierarchy of needs (in order of priority)
   a. Physiologic needs (oxygen and fluid sufficiency, healthful nutrition, normal body temperature and elimination patterns, adequate shelter and rest, sexual fulfillment)
   b. Safety and security (clothing, stable living environment, societal rules and laws)
   c. Love and belonging (relationships with family and friends)
   d. Self-esteem (control, respect, dignity, competence)
   e. Self-actualization (contentment, satisfaction)
3. Application to nursing
   a. Maslow's theory provides a framework for using the nursing process to meet client needs
   b. Nurses can use these needs to identify client problems (unmet needs) and formulate nursing diagnoses
   c. Nursing procedures help clients meet basic human needs

C. Nursing process
1. General information
   a. A series of planned steps directed toward a particular result
   b. Use of problem-solving techniques and the scientific method
2. Assessment
   a. Refers to the systematic and continuous collection, validation, and communication of client data
   b. Encompasses collection of subjective data (symptoms), which are experienced by the person affected and are obtained by the nursing history (interview), and objective data (signs), which can be verified by another person and are obtained by observation, measurement, auscultation, palpation, inspection, or percussion
3. Nursing diagnoses
   a. Consist of a two-part statement about the client's actual or potential health problems and their etiology, based on defining characteristics
   b. Are formulated by analyzing and interpreting assessment data and identifying the client's health problems, which a nurse, because of education and experience, is obligated to treat
   c. Are developed to focus nursing activities and plan nursing actions to resolve the client's health problems
   d. Involve the nurse's independent functions; the nurse is legally required by nurse practice acts to make nursing diagnoses and prescribe nursing actions
   e. Are based on the North American Nursing Diagnosis Association's (NANDA) standardized classification of nursing diagnoses, which promotes continuity throughout the profession
   f. Continue to be defined, classified, and described by NANDA, which was organized in 1982

4. Planning
   a. Involves developing the client's plan of care through setting priorities (establishing the preferred order of addressing the nursing diagnoses), writing client goals, and writing nursing actions (orders) to meet client goals
   b. Can use Maslow's hierarchy of needs or some other model or theory to set priorities; life-threatening problems always have the highest priority
   c. Necessitates identifying a client goal (the desired outcome after the nursing diagnosis is resolved); these goals should reflect the client's problems as described in the first part of the nursing diagnosis
   d. Requires inclusion of specific, behaviorally stated, measurable outcomes with the client goal so that evaluation can be completed
5. Implementation
   a. Refers to acting on the planned nursing orders and may involve carrying out independent, dependent, or interdependent actions
   b. Includes assessing the client before and after nursing actions and documenting the assessment and actions in the client's medical record
6. Evaluation
   a. Measures the extent to which the client's goals have been met
   b. Requires reexamination of assessment data, the nursing diagnosis, the goals, and nursing actions for possible revision if the client's goals are not met or only partially met

D. Nursing procedures
1. General information
   a. Consist of skilled nursing actions aimed at meeting the client's basic human needs
   b. Have common essential components — organization, client identification, client instruction, and use of the nursing process — that are addressed each time a nurse performs a procedure
2. Assessment
   a. Assess the need to carry out the procedure; if it is a dependent nursing action, read the physician's order sheet to ensure that a valid order has been written
   b. Evaluate the client's status before starting the procedure
   c. Determine the client's knowledge of the procedure, including why it is necessary and how the client participates in it
   d. Check the client's wristband to ensure proper identification
   e. Assess the client's mobility and ability to assist and cooperate with the procedure as necessary
3. Nursing diagnosis
   a. Interpret assessment data to identify the client's health problems and needs
   b. Develop appropriate nursing diagnoses based on assessment data

4. Planning
    a. Review the procedure in the institution's manual, and prepare for any procedural changes based on the client's needs
    b. Prepare a teaching plan for the client and family members, including information about the nature and purpose of the procedure; explain the client's role, including participation, if any
    c. Assemble needed supplies and equipment, taking into consideration the client's needs and the procedure itself
    d. Provide privacy by pulling curtains around the client's bed or closing the door to the room
5. Implementation
    a. Maintain surgical asepsis, with special emphasis on proper handwashing, and use proper body mechanics at all times
    b. Communicate with the client throughout the procedure, explaining each step and providing emotional support, as needed
    c. Perform the procedure according to the institution's performance criteria
    d. Dispose of or clean equipment and supplies in accordance with the nature of the procedure, type of equipment, and institution policies
    e. Record the client's status and the procedure's implementation and outcome legibly, promptly, completely, and accurately, using the appropriate documentation form
6. Evaluation
    a. Assess the client's tolerance of the procedure
    b. Decide whether the desired outcome has been attained and whether any undesirable effects have occurred
    c. Promote the client's comfort and cleanliness

Points to Remember

Nursing is a theory-based discipline.

The nursing process is a systematic, scientific method of planning and providing nursing care.

The five steps of the nursing process are assessment, diagnosis, planning, implementation, and evaluation.

Nursing procedures require specific actions to meet client needs.

All nursing procedures have common essential components, including organization, client identification, client instruction, and use of the nursing process.

Glossary

Assessment — first step of the nursing process, in which the nurse collects subjective and objective data

Client goal — component of the planning step of the nursing process that describes the desired outcome when the nursing diagnosis is resolved

Defining characteristics — assessment data that provide evidence of a client's health problem

Nursing action — component of the planning step of the nursing process, in which a nurse writes instructions for nursing care; also called a nursing order or nursing intervention

Nursing diagnosis — statement of actual or potential health problems that a nurse is legally required to treat

Nursing history — client or family interview conducted by a nurse on a client's admission to an institution to obtain information for beginning the nursing process

Assessing Vital Signs

Learning Objectives

After studying this section, the reader should be able to:

● Differentiate among oral, rectal, and axillary temperatures.

● List five commonly used pulse sites.

● Review the purpose of assessing each vital sign.

● Describe the procedures for assessing temperature, pulse, respirations, and blood pressure.

● Discuss the proper documentation of each vital sign.

II. Assessing Vital Signs

A. Introduction

1. Vital signs reflect the body's physiologic status and ability to regulate temperature, maintain local and systemic blood flow, and oxygenate tissues
2. Vital signs (also known as cardinal signs) include temperature, pulse, respirations, and blood pressure
3. Changes in vital signs can indicate sudden or gradual changes in the client's status; significant changes should be reported immediately to the charge nurse or physician
4. Vital signs can vary, depending on the time of day they are measured and on the client's condition, age, emotional status, exercise level, and food intake
5. Because of these variables, assessment of vital signs requires keen nursing judgment of the client and the situation
6. Vital signs are commonly assessed:
   a. On admission
   b. According to institution policy or physician's order, such as every 4 hours
   c. Before and after any invasive procedure, such as surgery
   d. Before and after administration of any medication that affects the cardiovascular or respiratory system
   e. When a client complains of any change in his condition, such as light-headedness or confusion
   f. When a client's condition worsens, as with a sudden increase in pain

B. Body temperature assessment

1. General information
   a. Body temperature records the balance between heat loss and heat production
   b. Assessing the body temperature reveals the core body temperature — that of the deep tissues or body interior
   c. Common sites for obtaining body temperature are the mouth, rectum, axilla, and ear (tympanic membrane)
   d. Three types of thermometer may be used to record body temperature: mercury-filled glass, electronic, and disposable chemical (disposable chemical thermometers are rarely used in institutions) (see *Comparing thermometer types*)
   e. Normal oral temperatures range from 97° to 99.5° F (36° to 37.5° C)
   f. Rectal temperatures are usually one degree higher than oral ones; axillary temperatures, one or two degrees lower
   g. Body temperature fluctuates with rest and activity; it is usually lowest during early morning hours and highest in late afternoon because of circadian rhythm

COMPARING THERMOMETER TYPES

TYPE	MECHANISM OF ACTION	ADVANTAGES	DISADVANTAGES
Mercury	Heat expands mercury	• Easy to store • Inexpensive • Readily available	• Accuracy varies despite manufacturers' efforts to standardize • Risk of breakage and cross contamination • Temperature recorded more slowly than with other thermometers • Mercury column can be difficult to read
Electronic	Heat alters the amount of current running through a reservoir	• Rapid recording and easy to read • Extremely accurate when properly charged and calibrated • Reduces risk of breakage • Easy to store • Eliminates risk of cross contamination	• Equipment is expensive (although nursing time saved may offset cost) • Recalibration required occasionally
Chemical	Heat initiates a chemical reaction	• Eliminates risk of cross contamination and breakage • Records temperature faster than mercury thermometer	• Improper storage may cause inaccuracy • Adapter needed for rectal use • Plastic strip in client's mouth may cause discomfort

h. Other factors affecting body temperature include *sex* (women normally have higher temperatures than men, especially during ovulation), *age* (temperature is highest in newborns and lowest in elderly persons), *emotions* (heightened emotions raise temperature, whereas depressed emotions lower it), and *external environment* (heat raises temperature while cold lowers it)

2. Purpose
   a. To obtain baseline data on admission to the hospital
   b. To guard against hyperthermia or hypothermia
   c. To monitor the client's response to a procedure or therapy
   d. To detect and follow the course of a febrile illness

3. Procedure: Taking oral temperature with a glass thermometer
   a. Determine when the client last ingested hot or cold fluids or smoked; wait 15 to 30 minutes before measuring the temperature

    b. Wash hands and rinse the thermometer thoroughly in cold water if it has been stored in disinfectant

    c. Check the reading by holding the thermometer horizontally at eye level and rotating it between the thumb and forefinger until the mercury line can be clearly seen

    d. If necessary, shake down the mercury by holding the thermometer between the thumb and forefinger at the end farthest from the bulb and sharply flicking the wrist down as though cracking a whip; repeat until the mercury is below 96° F (35.5° C)

    e. Gently place the thermometer under the client's tongue in the posterior sublingual pocket lateral to the center of the jaw; then ask the client to close his lips around the thermometer

    f. Leave the thermometer in place for 2 to 3 minutes or according to institution policy

    g. Remove the thermometer, wipe it with a tissue in a rotating motion from fingers toward the bulb, and read the temperature (to the nearest tenth of a degree)

    h. Wash the thermometer in tepid, soapy water, rinse in cool water, dry, and store

    i. Wash hands

4. Procedure: Taking oral temperature with an electronic thermometer

    a. Gather equipment: electronic thermometer, probe, and disposable probe covers

    b. Attach the oral probe (blue tip) to the unit

    c. Slide the disposable plastic probe cover over the thermometer probe until it is secure; do not put pressure on the tip (the ejection button)

    d. Gently place the probe under the client's tongue in the posterior sublingual pocket

    e. When the unit beeps (approximately 20 to 30 seconds after insertion), remove the thermometer probe and read the temperature on the digital display

    f. Push the ejection button to discard the probe cover into a trash receptacle, and return the electronic thermometer unit to the storage well for recharging

    g. Wash hands

5. Procedure: Taking rectal temperature

    a. Provide privacy for the client

    b. Wash hands and don clean disposable gloves

    c. Prepare a glass thermometer as suggested in procedure for oral temperature, or prepare an electronic thermometer using a red probe and probe cover

    d. Place the client in Sims' position, with the upper leg flexed, and fold bed linens to expose only the anal area

    e. Lubricate a glass thermometer or probe cover with a water-soluble lubricant

     f. Ask the client to take a deep breath; then gently insert the thermometer or covered probe into the anus toward the umbilicus, ½″ (1.3 cm) for an infant and 1½″ (3.8 cm) for an adult

     g. Hold the thermometer in place for 2 minutes or according to institution policy; hold an electronic thermometer in place until the unit beeps (about 15 to 20 seconds)

     h. Remove, read, and clean equipment as suggested for oral temperature

6. Procedure: Taking axillary temperature
   a. Provide privacy for the client
   b. Wash hands and prepare the glass or electronic thermometer as suggested in procedure for oral temperature
   c. Remove the client's gown to expose the axilla, and place the client in a supine or sitting position
   d. Place the thermometer bulb or the tip of the covered electronic probe into the center of the axilla
   e. Lower the client's arm over the thermometer, and place his forearm over his chest
   f. Leave a thermometer in place for 5 to 10 minutes; an electronic probe, until the unit beeps (remain with the patient at all times)
   g. Remove, read, and clean equipment as suggested for oral temperature

7. Documentation
   a. Record the client's temperature on a worksheet, graph, or flowsheet
   b. Indicate the site used and the time the temperature was taken
   c. Report any unusual findings to the charge nurse or physician

8. Nursing considerations
   a. Taking an oral temperature is contraindicated in a child younger than age 5 (who might bite down on a glass thermometer), in an irrational or unconscious client, in a client who has recently had oral surgery, and, in some institutions, in a client who is receiving oxygen or who has a tracheostomy
   b. Taking a rectal temperature is contraindicated in a client with rectal disease, one who has had rectal surgery, or one who may be at risk for rectal perforation from the thermometer
   c. Taking an axillary temperature is a safe, accessible, and easily tolerated alternative for a pediatric client
   d. Use the same thermometer for repeated temperature taking in a client to avoid variations caused by equipment differences
   e. Rinse mercury thermometers in cold water to prevent breakage
   f. Return electronic thermometers to their chargers so that they are ready for use when needed
   g. Never use an oral thermometer to take a rectal temperature; its long, slender bulb may puncture or injure rectal tissues
   h. Do not take an axillary temperature immediately after bathing the client's axilla; water temperature and friction of washing and drying can affect the client's body temperature

C. Pulse assessment

1. General information
   a. A client's pulse can be felt (palpated) peripherally or heard (auscultated) each time the heart's left ventricle contracts and forces blood into the aorta
   b. A *peripheral pulse* is a recurring fluid wave that courses through the arteries when blood is pumped into an already full aorta during ventricular contraction, flaring its walls
   c. An *apical pulse* is the sound heard during ventricular contraction
   d. Peripheral pulse sites are most easily palpated where an artery passes alongside or over a bone
   e. Common peripheral pulse sites are the temporal, carotid, brachial, radial, femoral, popliteal, dorsalis pedis, and posterior tibialis arteries; the radial pulse is the most commonly used peripheral pulse site for an adult (see *Pulse sites*)
   f. An apical pulse is taken by auscultating the apex of the heart with a stethoscope and counting the heart beats; used when an exact count is needed or when the client has an irregular heart rate or is younger than age 3
   g. An apical-radial pulse is taken by simultaneously counting the apical and radial beats; usually requires two nurses, one to auscultate the apical pulse and one to palpate the radial pulse
2. Assessment
   a. The client's pulse is assessed for rate (number of beats per minute), rhythm (pattern or regularity of the beats), and volume or amplitude (amount of blood pumped with each beat)
   b. Usually, an adult heart rate ranges from 60 to 80 beats/minute; slightly faster in women and older adults (70 to 80 beats/minute) and more rapid in children (90 to 140 beats/minute)
   c. *Tachycardia* (a heart rate greater than 100 beats/minute) can be caused by stress, hypoxia, strenuous (and usually infrequent) exercise, fever, hemorrhage, shock, and congestive heart disease
   d. *Bradycardia* (a heart rate less than 60 beats/minute) can be caused by moderate (and usually regular) exercise, certain drug therapies (such as digoxin), or a pathologic condition (such as increased intracranial pressure)
   e. Heart rhythm refers to the time interval between each heart beat
   f. A normal heart rhythm is described as regular; a consistently irregular rhythm, or *arrhythmia,* indicates heart malfunction
   g. The amplitude of a pulse can be described as *bounding* (pulse is felt by exerting only slight pressure over the artery) or *weak and thready* (pulse is difficult to feel or barely felt and easily obliterated with firm pressure)
   h. Doppler ultrasound equipment can be used to assess weak and thready pulses
3. Purpose
   a. To obtain a baseline measure of the client's heart rate and rhythm

PULSE SITES

PULSE	LOCATION
Apical	Auscultated at the apex of the heart; in an adult, on the left side of the chest, no more than 3″ (7.6 cm) to the left of the sternum, at the 4th or 5th intercostal space
Brachial	Palpated medially in the antecubital space (elbow crease) or at the inner aspect of the biceps muscle
Carotid	Palpated at the side of the neck, below the earlobe, under the mandible
Dorsalis pedis	Palpated along the top of the foot (pedal) over the instep
Femoral	Palpated midway between the anterior superior iliac spine and the symphysis pubis
Popliteal	Palpated in the popliteal fossa (knee crease)
Posterior tibialis	Palpated on the inner side of each ankle, below the medial malleolus
Radial	Palpated on the thumb side of the inner aspect of the wrist
Temporal	Palpated over the temporal bone of the skull, above and lateral to the eye

Temporal pulse
Carotid pulse
Brachial pulse
Radial pulse
Femoral pulse
Popliteal pulse
Dorsalis pedis
Posterior tibialis

b. To monitor changes in the client's cardiovascular status
c. To monitor the heart's response to a disease, procedure, or therapy (such as use of digoxin in a client with heart failure)
d. To assess blood flow to a specific body part
4. Procedure: Taking peripheral pulse
   a. Gather equipment: watch with a second hand
   b. Wash hands
   c. Help the client assume a comfortable position
   d. Place the fingertips of the middle two or three fingers along the appropriate artery and gently press
   e. Count the pulse for 1 minute (if the rhythm is regular, count the pulse for 30 seconds and multiply by 2)

5. Procedure: Taking apical pulse
   a. Gather equipment: stethoscope and watch with a second hand
   b. Clean the stethoscope's earpieces and diaphragm with an alcohol pad
   c. Place the client in a supine or sitting position
   d. Warm the stethoscope's diaphragm against the palm of the hand for a few seconds
   e. Move the client's gown to expose the chest
   f. Locate the pulse site on the left side of the chest, no more than 3" (8 cm) to the left of the sternum and under the 4th or 5th intercostal space
   g. Listen for heart sounds, which are heard as "lub-dub"
   h. Count the pulse for 1 minute (if the rhythm is regular, count the pulse for 30 seconds and multiply by 2); note any irregularities in rate or rhythm
6. Procedure: Taking apical-radial pulse
   a. Enlist the aid of another nurse
   b. Gather equipment: stethoscope and watch with a second hand
   c. Place the client in a supine position
   d. Locate apical and radial pulse sites
   e. Palpate the radial pulse for 60 seconds while the other nurse simultaneously auscultates the apical pulse
7. Documentation
   a. Record pulse site, heart rate and rhythm, and pulse amplitude
   b. Report any abnormalities to the charge nurse or physician
8. Nursing considerations
   a. When the peripheral pulse is irregular, take an apical pulse to measure heart beats more directly
   b. If a second nurse is unavailable to assist with an apical-radial pulse measurement, hold the stethoscope in place with the hand holding the watch and palpate the radial pulse with the other hand; feel for any discrepancies between the apical and radial pulses
   c. Compare the client's pulse rate and character with previous readings; if an apical pulse is taken, compare rates to detect any significant changes

D. Respiration assessment
1. General information
   a. Respiration—the process of oxygen intake and carbon dioxide output by the lungs—consists of *inhalation* and *exhalation*
   b. One inhalation and one exhalation count as one respiration
   c. The client should be at rest and unaware that a nurse is observing respirations
2. Assessment
   a. Respirations are assessed for rate, rhythm, depth, and character (see *Common respiratory patterns*)
   b. Respiratory rate refers to the number of breaths that a client takes each minute

COMMON RESPIRATORY PATTERNS

The chart below describes common respiratory patterns and their characteristics. To determine the rate, rhythm, and depth of a client's respirations, a nurse should observe him at rest, making sure he is unaware that his respirations are being counted. A person conscious of his respirations may alter his natural pattern. The nurse should count respirations for at least 1 minute. Counting for only a fraction of a minute and then multiplying can throw the count off by as much as 4 respirations/minute.

TYPE	CHARACTERISTICS
Eupnea	Normal respirations and rhythm. For adults and teenagers, 12 to 20 breaths/minute; ages 2 to 12, 20 to 30 breaths/minute; newborns, 30 to 50 breaths/minute.
Tachypnea	Increased respirations, as seen in fever. Respirations increase about 4 breaths/minute for every degree Fahrenheit above normal.
Bradypnea	Slower but regular respirations. Can occur when the brain's respiratory control center is affected by opiate narcotics, tumor, alcohol, metabolic disorder, or respiratory decompensation. Occurrence is normal during sleep.
Apnea	Absence of breathing; may be periodic.
Hyperpnea	Deeper respirations; rate normal.
Cheyne-Stokes	Respirations gradually become faster and deeper than normal, then slower, over 30 to 170 seconds. Alternate with periods of apnea that last 20 to 60 seconds.
Biot's	Faster and deeper respirations than normal, with abrupt pauses in between. Each breath has same depth; may occur with spinal meningitis or other central nervous system disorders.
Kussmaul's	Faster and deeper respirations without pauses. In adults, more than 20 breaths/minute. Breathing usually sounds labored, with deep breaths that resemble sighs; can occur from renal failure or metabolic acidosis.
Apneustic	Prolonged gasping inhalation, followed by extremely short, inefficient exhalation. Can occur from lesions in the brain's respiratory center.

    c. The normal respiratory rate is 12 to 20 breaths/minute in a resting adult; the rate is higher in infants and in those who are exercising, feeling stress, or suffering from certain diseases, such as infections or respiratory or cardiac disorders

    d. *Tachypnea* is an adult respiratory rate greater than 24 breaths/minute; *apnea* is the absence of respirations

    e. Rhythm refers to the regularity of inhalations and exhalations; diseases such as pneumonia can cause irregular respirations

    f. Depth is the volume of air inhaled and exhaled with each respiration and can be described as *normal, deep,* or *shallow*

    g. Abnormal characteristics include dyspnea (difficulty in breathing), orthopnea (difficulty in breathing unless sitting), wheezing (narrowing of airways, causing whistling or sighing sound), stridor (high-pitched sound heard on inhalation), rales (sound caused by air passing through fluid or mucus in the airways, usually on inhalation), and rhonchi (sound caused by air passing through airways narrowed by fluids, edema, or muscle spasm, usually during exhalation)

3. Purpose
    a. To obtain baseline data on respiratory rate and characteristics
    b. To monitor effects of pathologic conditions, such as infections, on the client's respirations
    c. To monitor the client's response to a specific therapy, such as oxygen or medication administration

4. Procedure: Assessing respirations
    a. Place a hand against the client's chest to feel its movements, or place the client's arm across his chest and observe chest movements while keeping fingers on the radial pulse, as if continuing to take the pulse
    b. Count respirations for 1 minute
    c. Observe chest movements to determine the depth of respiration
    d. Listen to the client's breathing for abnormal characteristics

5. Documentation
    a. Document the respiratory rate, depth, rhythm, and characteristics
    b. Report any significant change in rate, rhythm, or depth or any abnormal characteristics to the charge nurse or physician

6. Nursing considerations
    a. Count respirations after counting the pulse with the fingertips still on the client's artery
    b. Report rate changes that occur suddenly; a rate of fewer than 8 or more than 40 breaths/minute usually indicates a respiratory problem
    c. Observe the client for signs of dyspnea, such as anxious facial expression, flaring nostrils, or heaving chest wall

E. Blood pressure
1. General information
    a. Blood pressure — the force exerted by circulating blood against the arterial wall — consists of systolic and diastolic pressures

b. *Systolic* blood pressure is the highest pressure exerted when the left ventricle contracts (approximately 120 mm Hg in a healthy adult); reflects the integrity of the heart and arterial system

c. *Diastolic* blood pressure is the lowest pressure exerted when the left ventricle relaxes (approximately 80 mm Hg in a healthy adult); indicates vascular resistance

d. Normal blood pressure in an adult ranges from 110/60 to 140/90 mm Hg; hypertension, or high blood pressure, is persistent blood pressure readings above 140/90 mm Hg

e. Factors that can decrease blood pressure include age (infants have the lowest blood pressure), drugs (such as antihypertensives, narcotic analgesics, general anesthetics, and diuretics), and loss of blood volume (such as in hemorrhaging or severely burned clients)

f. Factors that can increase blood pressure include age (blood pressure rises with age), exercise, increased blood volume, fear, anxiety, pain, vasoconstricting drugs (such as epinephrine), high sodium intake, arteriosclerosis, renal disease, smoking, and obesity

g. Blood pressure is measured with a sphygmomanometer, blood pressure cuff, and stethoscope

2. Purpose
   a. To obtain a baseline blood pressure measurement
   b. To assess the client's cardiovascular status
   c. To assess the client's response to blood or fluid volume loss after surgery, childbirth, trauma, or burns
   d. To evaluate the client's response to changes in his condition after treatment with fluids, medications, or other therapies

3. Procedure: Auscultating blood pressure
   a. Gather equipment: stethoscope and sphygmomanometer with a blood pressure cuff of appropriate size (4¾" to 5½" [12 to 14 cm] wide for average adult arm; narrower for infants, children, and adults with thin arms; 7" to 8" [18 to 20 cm] for obese clients or to use for leg pressure readings)
   b. Wash hands
   c. Help the client assume a comfortable lying or sitting position, with the arm to be wrapped supported at heart level
   d. Wrap the cuff smoothly and snugly above the upper part of the arm so that the cuff's lower edge is about 1" to 2" (2.5 to 5 cm) above the antecubital space, with the center of the cuff's bladder over the brachial artery
   e. Fasten the cuff securely, or tuck in the end of the cuff
   f. Palpate the brachial pulse with fingertips
   g. Tighten the screw valve on the air pump and inflate the cuff while palpating the artery; note when the pulse disappears
   h. Deflate the cuff by loosening the screw valve, note when the pulse reappears, deflate the cuff fully, and wait 30 seconds

     i. Place the diaphragm of the stethoscope over the brachial artery, and inflate the cuff 30 mm Hg above the point at which the pulse disappeared

     j. Gradually open the release valve, allowing mercury to fall slowly; note the point at which the first clear sound is heard (this first Korotkoff sound indicates the systolic pressure)

     k. Listen for the point at which the sound becomes muffled (fourth Korotkoff sound) and the point at which the last sound is heard (this fifth Korotkoff sound indicates the diastolic pressure)

     l. Completely deflate the cuff and remove it from the client's arm

     m. Wash hands

4. Procedure: Palpating blood pressure
    a. Apply a blood pressure cuff, following the same steps as for auscultating blood pressure
    b. Palpate the brachial or radial artery with the fingertips of one hand
    c. Inflate the cuff to a pressure 30 mm Hg above the point at which the pulse disappears
    d. Slowly deflate the cuff; as soon as the pulse is palpable, note the sphygmomanometer reading (this reading is the "palpated systolic pressure")
    e. Deflate the cuff completely, and remove it from the client's arm

5. Documentation
    a. Document the blood pressure reading and site according to institution policy on the worksheet and the client's record
    b. Chart the two pressures; for example, 120/80, where 120 is the systolic and 80 the diastolic (the American Heart Association recommends that the first muffled sound be used as the diastolic reading in children and that the last sound heard be recorded as the diastolic reading in adults)
    c. Record the palpated blood pressure; for example, *90 palpable*
    d. Report significant changes to the charge nurse or physician

6. Nursing considerations
    a. Avoid taking blood pressure readings in an arm that is injured or diseased, is on the same side as past breast surgery, has an intravenous or arteriovenous shunt, or is wrapped in a bulky bandage or cast
    b. Be sure the sphygmomanometer is at eye level for accurate blood pressure readings
    c. Do not reinflate the cuff without completely deflating it and waiting at least 30 seconds
    d. If the client's blood pressure is 30 mm Hg or more below baseline, retake the reading in the other arm, and assess for signs and symptoms of hypotension (such as changes in pulse, respirations, or temperature), shock, or hemorrhage
    e. If no other supporting data are available, retake the blood pressure 15 to 30 minutes later; if other signs of distress are seen, place the client in a supine position, report to the charge nurse or physician, and continue to monitor the client closely

f. If the client's blood pressure is 30 mm Hg or more above baseline, retake the reading in the other arm, and assess for signs and symptoms of hypertension, headache, confusion, chest pain, or difficult breathing

g. If the client's blood pressure is difficult or impossible to auscultate, assess the pulse and respirations and check proper functioning of the equipment; instruct the client to raise his arm above his shoulder while the cuff is rapidly inflated, then lower the arm and take the reading; try the procedure on the other arm or wait and repeat on the same arm; measure by palpation if blood pressure still cannot be auscultated

Points to Remember

Vital signs reflect the body's physiologic status.

Changes in vital signs may indicate changes in the client's health, and significant changes should be reported immediately to the charge nurse or physician.

An oral temperature is contraindicated in a young child, in an irrational or unconscious client, and in a client who has recently had mouth surgery.

An apical pulse is indicated in a client with an irregular heart rate and in infants and young children.

Avoid taking blood pressure readings in an arm that is injured or diseased, is on the same side as breast surgery, has an intravenous or arteriovenous shunt, or is wrapped in a bulky bandage or cast.

Glossary

Apnea – absence of respirations

Bradycardia – slow heart rate, usually fewer than 60 beats/minute in an adult

Circadian rhythm – 24-hour cycle during which certain phenomena in living organisms occur at about the same time each day

Core temperature – temperature of the deep tissues and body interior

Hypertension – high blood pressure, usually greater than 140/90 mm Hg in an adult

Tachycardia – rapid heart rate, usually greater than 100 beats/minute in an adult

Tachypnea – rapid respiratory rate, usually greater than 24 breaths/minute in an adult at rest

Maintaining Asepsis

Learning Objectives

After studying this section, the reader should be able to:

- Identify the six components of the infection chain.

- Differentiate between medical and surgical asepsis.

- Discuss various medical aseptic practices.

- Explain the universal precautions for client care.

- Describe procedures used to ensure medical and surgical asepsis.

III. Maintaining Asepsis

A. Introduction

1. Asepsis is the absence of infection or of germs or pathogens (disease-producing microorganisms) that cause infection
2. An infection results from the actions of pathogens within the body and involves a cyclical interaction of six components (infectious agent, reservoir, mode of transmission, portal of exit, susceptible host, and portal of entry), collectively called the *infection chain* (see *Infection chain*)
3. Aseptic technique refers to practices or procedures used by nurses and other health care professionals to help prevent infection or interrupt the infection chain
4. Asepsis is classified as medical or surgical
   a. *Medical asepsis,* or clean technique, involves practices or procedures that reduce the number and transmission of pathogens
   b. In medical asepsis, an article becomes contaminated (unclean, not to be used by another person until cleaned or disinfected) when it is touched by the client or his used supplies
   c. *Surgical asepsis,* or sterile technique, involves practices or procedures that render and keep objects and areas free of all pathogens
   d. In surgical asepsis, an article becomes contaminated (unsterile) when it is touched by an unsterile object
5. Pathogens are destroyed by *disinfection* (a process that destroys pathogens on articles) or *sterilization* (a process by which all microorganisms, including spores, are destroyed)
6. Disinfection and sterilization can be accomplished by physical methods (steam, boiling water, dry heat, and radiation) or chemical methods (ethylene oxide gas or chemical solutions of chlorine compounds, iodine, and alcohol)

B. Medical asepsis

1. General information
   a. Hospitalized clients are especially susceptible to infections because of lowered resistance from illness, medication, or therapy; increased exposure to pathogens; and invasive procedures performed in the hospital
   b. Medical aseptic practices are used for all clients in the hospital to prevent the spread of infection (see *Practices of medical asepsis,* page 28)
   c. In the United States, the Centers for Disease Control (CDC) provides guidelines for medical aseptic practices and isolation techniques; these guidelines are considered minimum protection standards, and institutions can modify them to meet specific needs
   d. Medical aseptic practices include personal hygiene, such as handwashing after use of the toilet; specific hospital practices, such as not placing soiled linens on the floor; and special methods of medical asepsis used to isolate and prevent the spread of pathogens

INFECTION CHAIN

The infection chain has six components: infectious agent, reservoir, mode of transmission, portal of exit, susceptible host, and portal of entry. Infection control procedures attempt to break the chain by eliminating or minimizing one or more of these components.

The agent must have a reservoir (such as water, fluids, or human tissue) in which to grow and must be able to leave the reservoir through a portal of exit, such as the gastrointestinal, respiratory, or genitourinary tract.

The mode of transmission bridges the gap between the agent and its host by *contact* (touching an infected site or person or an inanimate object contaminated by an infected person), a *common vehicle* (such as a multidose medication vial, a contaminated needle, or blood), a *vector* (transmitted by a nonhuman carrier, such as an insect or animal), or an *airborne contaminant* (such as contacting or inhaling droplets from a person who has sneezed).

The host is infected when the agent traverses his defenses through a portal of entry, such as a natural body orifice (nose, mouth, anus), any skin break, or placement of an invasive device into a body orifice or artificial opening.

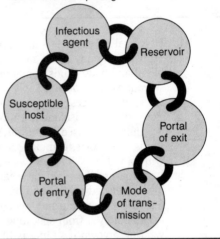

    e. Handwashing is the most effective way to prevent the spread of pathogens and interrupt the infection chain

2. Isolation techniques

    a. Special methods of medical asepsis, called isolation techniques or practices, are used in health care facilities

    b. Isolation techniques are categorized by type of disease (disease specific), method of transmission (category specific), and type of precautions needed to protect health care workers from potentially infected blood and body fluids (universal precautions or body substance isolation)

    c. In 1983, the CDC revised its guidelines to include disease-specific isolation, which identifies precautions for each disease, and category-specific isolation, which identifies precautions for each category

    d. Category-specific isolation consists of measures taken to interfere with the mode of transmission and includes strict contact, respiratory, enteric, drainage, and blood and body fluid precautions

    e. In 1987, in response to the danger of acquired immunodeficiency syndrome (AIDS) transmission in hospitals, the CDC formulated universal precautions, which state that health care workers should consider all clients potentially infected with AIDS and other bloodborne pathogens

PRACTICES OF MEDICAL ASEPSIS

● Keep soiled articles, linens, and equipment from touching the uniform.
● Do not place any equipment, supplies, or soiled items on the floor.
● Do not shake linens or raise dust.
● Clean the least soiled area first, the most soiled area last.
● Pour liquids into the sink close to the drain to avoid splattering.
● Follow institution or Centers for Disease Control guidelines for isolation techniques.

    f. Universal precautions — infection-control guidelines based on risk of exposure to body fluids rather than on the diagnosed disease — apply to blood and body fluids containing visible blood, semen, or vaginal secretions; they do not apply to nasal secretions, sputum, saliva, sweat, tears, urine, feces, or vomitus unless blood is visible

    g. Body substance isolation, a more inclusive variation of universal precautions, is used for all clients and includes precautions for all body fluids, secretions, and excretions, whether or not they are contaminated with blood

    h. Isolation practices include wearing clean disposable gloves when handling blood and body fluids and discarding gloves after one use; wearing masks for some category-specific groups or wearing nonpermeable masks to protect eyes from splashing of blood (discarded after one use); and wearing a gown if soiling is likely or wearing a nonpermeable gown when splashing of blood is likely

3. Purpose
    a. To prevent transfer of pathogens to health care workers, other clients, and visitors
    b. To reduce the number of pathogens and confine them to a specific area or room

4. Procedure: Handwashing
    a. Assemble equipment: liquid soap (recommended) or bar soap, running tap water, paper towels, and orangewood stick (optional)
    b. Stand in front of the sink but do not allow the uniform to touch the sink or become wet, either of which will contaminate the uniform
    c. Remove jewelry (in some institutions, a plain wedding band is permitted); do not wear fingernail polish
    d. Turn on the water and adjust its force; regulate temperature until the water is warm
    e. Wet the hands and wrist area, keeping the hands lower than the elbows to allow water to flow to the fingertips
    f. Use about 1 teaspoon of liquid soap or lather thoroughly with bar soap; after washing, rinse the bar and return it to the soap dish
    g. With firm rubbing and circular motions, wash the palms and backs of the hands, each finger and between the fingers, knuckles, wrists, and forearms at least as far up as contamination is likely to occur

h. Continue washing for 30 seconds
i. Use fingernails of the other hand or an orangewood stick to clean under the fingernails
j. Rinse thoroughly under running water with the fingers pointed downward, and dry the hands, wrists, and forearms well with paper towels
k. Turn off the faucet, using a paper towel
5. Procedure: Removing clean disposable gloves
   a. Grasping the outside of one glove with the fingers of the opposite gloved hand, remove the first glove, turning it inside out
   b. Place the removed glove in the palm of the gloved hand
   c. Place several fingers of the ungloved hand inside the remaining glove, and turn the glove inside out over the palm
   d. Discard both gloves into a lined trash container
   e. Wash hands
6. Procedure: Donning and removing an isolation gown
   a. Review institution policy or CDC guidelines to determine the need for a gown
   b. Grasp the top of the gown from the inside, keeping the outside facing away from the body
   c. Slide both arms forward through the sleeves until cuffs cover the wrists; tie the gown at the waist and neck
   d. Give client care as indicated
   e. Untie the waist ties and wash hands; then untie the neck ties and remove the gown without touching the outside
   f. Turn the gown inside out so that contaminated sides face each other, and discard it into the linen bag
7. Procedure: Applying and removing a mask
   a. Review institution policy or CDC guidelines to determine the need for a mask
   b. Apply the mask to the face and tie it securely
   c. Give client care as indicated
   d. Untie the mask, handling it by the strings
   e. Discard it into a lined trash container
   f. Wash hands
8. Procedure: Removing soiled linens and emptying trash
   a. Before leaving the isolation room, gather soiled linen and trash bags and take them to the door
   b. Ask an assistant to stand just outside the door while holding a clean bag, with hands protected under the bag's cuffed edge
   c. Place the soiled linen into the clean bag; then place trash bags into a second bag held by the assistant
   d. Have the assistant seal and label the bags according to institution policy
   e. Take the bags to an appropriate area for safe disposal

9. Documentation
   a. Document the type of isolation precautions used; do not document isolation precautions (such as handwashing or donning clean gloves) that are standard protocol for all clients
   b. Record the client's response to isolation practices
10. Nursing considerations
   a. Wash the hands after any prolonged contact with the client; before and after wearing gloves; after handling blood, other body fluids, secretions, or excretions; after contact with mucous membranes; or after handling contaminated dressings or equipment, such as bedpans
   b. Scrub the hands for 10 to 30 seconds before and after giving client care when contamination is minimal; scrub the hands for 1 to 4 minutes when they are visibly soiled
   c. Assemble all equipment before entering the client's room to reduce unnecessary handwashing and donning of gloves and gowns
   d. Do not touch the nose, mouth, or eyes when wearing gloves
   e. Wear one pair of gloves for each client
   f. Don gloves after putting on a gown and mask, if necessary; remove and discard them before removing a gown and mask

C. Surgical asepsis
1. General information
   a. Surgical asepsis is used in the operating room, delivery room, and certain diagnostic areas, such as the cystoscopy room
   b. A nurse uses surgical asepsis at the client's bedside whenever a procedure involves entering a sterile body cavity (such as the bladder), breaking skin integrity for an injection, or caring for a wound
   c. Sterile technique practices are followed when using surgical asepsis (see *Principles of sterile technique*)
   d. Sterile technique involves using a *sterile field,* which consists of a sterile tray or surface draped with a sterile towel or wrapper
2. Purpose
   a. To prevent introduction of microorganisms into the body
   b. To prevent infection of wounds
3. Procedure: Donning sterile gloves
   a. Wash the hands
   b. Place the sterile package on a clean, dry surface above the waist
   c. Open the outside wrapper and remove the inner package; then open the inner package and expose the gloves with cuffs toward you
   d. With one hand, grasp the edge of the folded cuff of one glove and slip the fingers of the opposite hand inside the glove
   e. Pull the glove on by holding onto the folded cuff
   f. Slip the gloved fingers under the cuff of the other glove, holding the thumb outward; then lift the glove upward, away from the wrapper
   g. Pull the glove onto the ungloved hand
   h. Adjust the gloves on both hands as needed

PRINCIPLES OF STERILE TECHNIQUE

• Use a sterile object to touch another sterile object to avoid contamination.
• Hold sterile objects above waist level.
• Keep the sterile field within sight.
• Avoid talking, coughing, sneezing, or reaching over the sterile field.

• Consider the 1″ (2.5 cm) edge of the sterile field contaminated.
• Do not spill solution on the sterile field cloth because moisture penetrating the cloth carries microorganisms to the sterile field by capillary action.

---

      i. Touch only the sterile area or sterile objects with the gloves

4. Procedure: Removing sterile gloves
   a. Grasping the outside of one glove with fingers of the opposite gloved hand, remove the first glove, turning it inside out
   b. Place the removed glove in the palm of the gloved hand
   c. Slide fingers of the ungloved hand inside the remaining glove, and remove the glove by turning it inside out over the palm
   d. Discard both gloves in an appropriate container
   e. Wash hands

5. Procedure: Preparing a sterile field
   a. Assemble supplies: package or tray containing sterile items specific to the procedure, sterile container, sterile solution, and sterile gloves
   b. Wash hands thoroughly
   c. Place the sealed sterile package containing sterile items on a clean, flat work surface above waist level
   d. Remove the outer plastic wrap: open the outermost flap away from the body, open side flaps, then open the last flap toward the body, touching only the outside of the package
   e. Use the opened wrapper as a sterile field

6. Procedure: Adding a sterile item to a sterile field
   a. Open the sterile item while holding the outside of the wrapper
   b. Peel the wrapper back over the hand
   c. Place the item onto the field at an angle without touching the wrapper to the field or reaching over the field
   d. Discard the wrapper

7. Procedure: Adding a sterile solution to a sterile container
   a. Remove the cap from the bottle of solution, and place it on a clean surface inside up
   b. Hold the bottle with the label in the palm of the hand
   c. Pour a small amount of liquid into a plastic-lined waste receptacle
   d. Slowly pour solution into the sterile container, holding the bottle directly above the container
   e. Replace the cap on the bottle

8. Procedure: Transferring items with forceps to a sterile field
   a. Open packages containing forceps and items to be added to the sterile field

    b. Grasp forceps handles and raise the instrument above waist level and away from the body

    c. With the ends of the forceps, grasp the item to be placed on the sterile field

    d. Raise the item straight up and lift it over and onto the sterile field, keeping the forceps handles outside the field

9. Documentation

    a. Document the procedure, noting that it was performed using sterile technique

    b. Do not document specific aspects of sterile technique, such as setting up a sterile field or donning and removing gloves

10. Nursing considerations

    a. If any portion of a sterile object touches an unsterile object, the entire field is contaminated and a new field must be set up

    b. Avoid talking over a sterile field; air currents contain microorganisms

    c. Use sterile technique for wound care, breaks in skin integrity, and procedures that involve entering a sterile cavity, such as the bladder

    d. Consider an article contaminated if uncertain of its sterility

Points to Remember

The infection chain consists of six components and can be interrupted by aseptic practices.

Medical aseptic practices are used for all clients to prevent the spread of infection.

Medical asepsis, or clean technique, includes any practices or procedures that reduce the number and transmission of pathogens.

Surgical asepsis, or sterile technique, includes any practices that render and maintain objects and areas free of microorganisms.

Hospitalized clients are especially susceptible to infection because of lowered resistance from illness, medication, or therapy; increased exposure to infection; and invasive procedures performed in the hospital.

Surgical asepsis is used in the operating room, delivery room, and certain diagnostic areas and when caring for clients with loss of skin integrity, giving injections, or entering a sterile cavity.

Glossary

Asepsis — absence of infection or of disease-producing microorganisms that cause infection

Disinfection — process that destroys pathogens on articles

Infection — invasion of the body by a pathogen, producing signs of disease

Pathogen — infectious agent (microorganism) capable of producing disease

Spores — reproductive unit of some lower organisms, such as fungi; a form assumed by certain bacteria resistant to heat, drying, and chemicals

Sterile field — work area free of microorganisms that is used to hold sterile items

Sterilization — process by which all microorganisms, including spores, are destroyed

Promoting Hygiene and Comfort

Learning Objectives

After studying this section, the reader should be able to:

• List three types of bath for a hospitalized client.

• Review the procedure for a complete bed bath.

• Discuss the procedure for mouth care in conscious and unconscious clients.

• Explain the purpose of a back rub.

• List the three types of bedmaking and their purpose.

IV. Promoting Hygiene and Comfort

A. Introduction
1. Personal hygiene refers to measures that promote personal cleanliness and grooming
   a. Hygiene is a basic need for a client's well-being and self-esteem
   b. Hygiene is also necessary for infection control
2. Hygienic practices are highly individualized and can be influenced by the client's:
   a. Culture
   b. Socioeconomic status
   c. Religion
   d. Developmental level
   e. Health status
   f. Personal preference
3. The nurse must be knowledgeable about these factors to provide individualized client care
4. The nurse assists the client in meeting hygiene needs by providing care that the client alone cannot or should not provide
5. The nurse should encourage the client to meet personal hygiene needs when possible

B. Bathing
1. General information
   a. The nurse provides cleansing or therapeutic baths
   b. Cleansing baths include a complete bed bath, a partial bed bath, and a tub bath or shower
   c. A *complete bed bath* consists of washing a dependent client's entire body in bed; a *complete bed bath with assistance* involves helping the client to wash (for example, the nurse washes the back or feet and legs)
   d. A *partial bed bath* consists of washing only parts of the client's body (such as feet or buttocks) that may cause discomfort or odor if left unwashed
   e. A *tub bath* or *shower* provides a more thorough cleansing than a bed bath; the amount of nursing assistance is determined by the client's age and health and by safety considerations
   f. A therapeutic bath is ordered by a physician for a specific purpose (see Moist Heat and Moist Cold, Section XI, for more information)
   g. Therapeutic baths include a *sitz bath* (to reduce inflammation and clean the perineal and perianal area), a *tepid sponge bath* (to reduce fever), and a *medicated tub bath* (to relieve skin irritation)
2. Purpose
   a. To clean the skin
   b. To provide comfort and relaxation
   c. To stimulate circulation
   d. To remove secretions and excretions

    e. To provide time for client assessment and teaching
    f. To allow inspection of the body for skin breakdown
3. Procedure: Giving a complete bed bath
    a. Gather equipment: two bath towels, two washcloths, soap, soap dish, emollient (if necessary), bath blanket, bedpan or urinal, wash basin, bed linen, laundry bag or cart, clean disposable gloves, and such personal supplies as lotion, deodorant, and toothbrush
    b. Provide privacy for the client, and offer him a bedpan or urinal
    c. Raise the bed to the highest position
    d. Remove bed linen; fold bed linen to be reused over a chair, and place soiled linen in a laundry bag
    e. Assist the client with oral hygiene
    f. Fill a wash basin two-thirds full with warm water, adding emollient, if necessary; use a thermometer to confirm that water temperature is 109° to 115° F (43° to 46° C); change water as necessary during the bath
    g. Place the client in a comfortable position (usually supine or semi-Fowler's), and remove his gown, maintaining privacy by covering him with a bath blanket; lay a bath towel over the client's chest
    h. Fold a washcloth on your hand like a mitt, with no loose ends
    i. Wash the client's eyes with warm water, using a separate portion of the washcloth for each eye and wiping from the inner to outer canthus; dry eyes gently but thoroughly
    j. Ask the client if he wants his face cleaned with soap; then wash, rinse, and dry the face, neck, and ears
    k. Place a bath towel lengthwise under the client's arm; wash the arm with soap and water, using long firm strokes from the fingers to the axilla (distal to proximal); rinse, dry well, and repeat for the other arm
    l. Apply deodorant or talcum powder if the client prefers
    m. Place the wash basin on a towel on the bed, and immerse the client's hands; help the client wash, rinse, and dry both hands
    n. Place a towel over the client's chest, and fold a bath blanket down to the pubic area; wash, rinse, and dry the chest and abdomen, taking special care to wash the skinfolds of a woman's breasts
    o. Cover the chest, abdomen, opposite leg, and perineum with a bath blanket; then slide a towel under the leg to be washed first
    p. Place the wash basin on the bed, next to the client's foot; bend the leg at the knee and immerse the foot in the basin; allow the foot to soak while washing the leg
    q. Wash the leg from ankle to knee and from knee to thigh, using long, firm, smooth strokes; rinse and dry well
    r. Wash and dry the foot, making sure to wash and dry thoroughly between the toes; wash the other leg and foot in the same manner
    s. Cover the client with the bath blanket, change the water, and place the client in a prone or sidelying position; place a towel lengthwise along the client's back and buttocks

     t. Wash, rinse, and dry the back from neck to buttocks, paying special attention to the folds of the anus and buttocks

     u. Give the client a back rub

     v. Place the client in a supine position and cover him with a bath blanket, placing one corner between the client's legs, one corner pointing to each side of the bed, and one corner over the client's chest

     w. Put on gloves

     x. Change water and use a clean washcloth to wash, rinse, and dry the perineum from front to back, paying special attention to skinfolds

     y. Discard gloves and help the client put on a clean gown or pajamas; comb the client's hair, and allow a female client to put on makeup

     z. Make the client's bed, place soiled linen in a laundry bag, then wash hands

4. Procedure: Giving a partial bed bath
   a. Help the client to the toilet or commode if permitted
   b. Follow the procedure for a complete bed bath
   c. Assist the client with washing arms, chest, legs, and feet

5. Procedure: Giving a tub bath or shower
   a. Ensure that the tub or shower is unoccupied, and check for cleanliness; clean according to institution policy
   b. Gather supplies: two towels, two washcloths, and personal care items
   c. Place a rubber mat or towel in the bottom of a tub or shower without a nonskid surface
   d. For a bath, fill the tub halfway with warm water (109° to 115° F [43° to 46° C]), checking temperature with a bath thermometer; for a shower, help the client to the shower room and assist as necessary, such as by adjusting the temperature or water flow or washing the client's back
   e. Instruct the client on the use of safety bars when getting in and out of the tub or shower and use of a call signal to summon help
   f. Help the client into the tub or shower
   g. Stay just outside the door in case the client needs assistance
   h. Drain the tub before the client gets out to minimize the risk of falling
   i. Help the client out of the tub or shower, and assist the client in drying and putting on a clean gown or pajamas
   j. Accompany the client back to the room and provide a back rub
   k. Clean the tub or shower according to institution policy
   l. Place soiled linen in a laundry bag; then wash hands

6. Documentation
   a. Document the type of bath given; some institutions include daily bath on a checklist
   b. Record the client's response to the bath
   c. Note the condition of the client's skin and any unusual findings, such as reddened areas, breaks in skin integrity, or rash

7. Nursing considerations
   a. Determine which type of bath is most appropriate before bathing a client

b. Inquire about the client's usual hygiene practices or preferences to individualize care
c. Identify factors that may put a client at risk for loss of skin integrity, such as immobility, reduced sensation, or poor circulation
d. Check the client during the bath for signs of skin problems, such as rash, redness, dryness, or breakdown
e. For some clients, such as those who are obese, wash the breasts and abdomen separately, paying special attention to skinfolds

C. Perineal care
1. General information
   a. Perineal care consists of washing the client's external genitalia and surrounding skin
   b. Perineal care is routinely performed when bathing any client and is provided more frequently to a client with an indwelling urinary catheter or perineal infection or after perineal or anal surgery or childbirth
2. Purpose
   a. To promote comfort and cleanliness
   b. To promote healing after surgery or childbirth
   c. To prevent infection in a client with an indwelling urinary catheter
3. Procedure: Giving perineal care
   a. Assemble equipment: wash basin, soap, soap dish, washcloths, towels, bath blanket, solution bottle, pitcher or container filled with warm water or prescribed solution, bedpan, perineal pad if necessary, and clean disposable gloves
   b. Explain the procedure and its purpose to the client
   c. Provide privacy, and drape the client with one corner of the bath blanket between the legs, one corner over the chest, and side corners around the feet, covering the legs
   d. Fill the wash basin with warm water at the appropriate temperature (usually 109° to 115° F [43° to 46° C]), and put on gloves
   e. Wash the upper and inner thighs with soap and water; dry thoroughly
   f. Place a female client on a bedpan, and clean the labia majora; spread the labia and wash around the clitoris, labia minora, and vagina from pubis to rectum, using a separate section of the washcloth for each stroke
   g. Pour warm water or a prescribed solution over the labia so that runoff drips into the bedpan, and dry the labia with a towel; help the client to a sidelying position and adjust the bath blanket
   h. Wash, rinse, and dry the male perineum and penis, using firm strokes; retract the foreskin of an uncircumsized male before cleaning, and replace after washing; wash the tip of the penis and shaft with firm, downward strokes; wash, rinse, and dry the scrotum
   i. Clean the anal area, first wiping off feces with toilet tissue, then wash, rinse, and dry, wiping from front to back
   j. Rinse washcloths and place soiled linen in a laundry bag

       k. Empty water and clean the wash basin with soap and water; rinse, dry, and return it to the client's storage area

       l. Discard gloves, help the client to a comfortable position, and remove the bath blanket

      m. Wash hands

   4. Documentation

       a. Record any significant problems, such as redness, excoriation, or swelling

       b. Note the amount, color, and odor of any discharge

       c. Document the client's tolerance of the procedure

   5. Nursing considerations

       a. Always use a front-to-back wiping motion for perineal care

       b. Apply a perineal pad when drainage or bleeding occurs

D. Mouth care

   1. General information

       a. The mouth can become excessively dry or irritated or can develop foul-tasting secretions (sordes) from illness or certain therapies

       b. Mouth care is usually part of bathing but is done more frequently if a client's condition warrants

       c. Frequency of mouth care is determined by the condition of the client's mouth and comfort level; it may be required as often as every 1 to 2 hours

       d. The nurse assists a conscious client and provides the mouth care for an unconscious client, making sure the client does not aspirate

   2. Purpose

       a. To clean the mouth and teeth as part of a personal hygiene routine

       b. To remove secretions from an unconscious client's mouth

       c. To maintain intact, well-hydrated mucosa

   3. Procedure: Performing mouth care for a conscious client

       a. Assess the client's ability to brush the teeth and rinse the mouth

       b. Gather equipment: toothpaste, toothbrush, water, emesis basin, towel, mouthwash, and dental floss; place on an overbed table

       c. Place a towel under the client's chin; wash hands and don clean disposable gloves if providing the mouth care

       d. Hold the toothbrush over the emesis basin, pour a small amount of water over it, and apply toothpaste

       e. Brush the client's teeth gently to avoid injuring the gums

       f. Allow the client to rinse with several sips of water and to swish and spit into the emesis basin

       g. Offer mouthwash and dental floss

       h. Help the client to wipe the mouth

       i. Remove and clean the emesis basin

       j. Wipe off the overbed table, place the soiled towel in a laundry bag, and remove and discard gloves; return equipment to its proper place

       k. Wash hands

4. Procedure: Performing mouth care for a client with dentures
   a. Gather equipment: toothbrush, toothpaste, fresh water or mouthwash, sink or emesis basin, gauze pad or washcloth, denture cup, denture cream or powder, towel, and clean disposable gloves; place on an overbed table
   b. Wash hands and put on gloves
   c. Ask the client to remove all dentures and place them in the denture cup; if the client cannot do this, use a gauze pad or washcloth to grasp the front of the upper denture with a thumb and forefinger, pull downward to break the suction, lift the lower denture, and place both dentures in the denture cup
   d. Fill a sink or emesis basin with water, cleaning the dentures over the water to prevent breakage if they fall
   e. Brush dentures on all surfaces with toothbrush and toothpaste; then rinse with tepid water
   f. Return dentures to the client, or store in the denture cup
   g. Have the client rinse and then gently brush the gums and tongue with a soft toothbrush
   h. Reinsert dentures (or allow the client to do so), inserting moistened upper denture first and pressing in place
   i. Remove and discard gloves, and clean and store supplies
   j. Wash hands
5. Procedure: Performing mouth care for an unconscious client
   a. Gather equipment: soft toothbrush, toothpaste, emesis basin, clean disposable gloves, water, towel, mouthwash, sponge toothbrush (Toothette) or padded tongue blades, irrigating syringe with rubber tip (optional), cleansing agent, lubricating jelly, and suction apparatus with catheter (optional)
   b. Wash hands and don gloves
   c. Position the client on one side, with the head lowered and tilted toward the mattress
   d. Place a towel and emesis basin under the client's chin
   e. Open the client's mouth and gently insert a padded tongue blade between the back molars
   f. Clean the teeth, gums, tongue, and inside cheeks with a soft toothbrush or moistened padded tongue blade; if necessary, have a second nurse suction as secretions accumulate
   g. Rinse with a moistened clean swab, Toothette, or irrigating syringe, repeating several times; allow for returned drainage or use suction; remove padded tongue blade
   h. Apply a thin layer of lubricating jelly to the client's lips
   i. Remove and discard gloves; clean equipment
   j. Return the client to an appropriate position
   k. Wash hands

6. Documentation
    a. Record mouth care on the appropriate form; some institutions include mouth care on a checklist
    b. Document any significant problems, such as ulcerations, lesions, swelling, bleeding, secretions, or pain
7. Nursing considerations
    a. Teach the client proper care of teeth during mouth care procedure
    b. Inspect the client's mouth and gums for ulcerations, lesions, bleeding, and secretions, and note any client complaints of pain
    c. Administer mouth care to a client receiving nothing by mouth as frequently as needed to keep the mouth moist and clean
    d. Consider the client's developmental level, preferences, and health status when planning frequency of mouth care and amount of assistance needed

E. Back rub
1. General information
    a. A back rub typically consists of massaging the back, shoulders, and lower neck
    b. A back rub is commonly scheduled after a client's bath or when preparing a client for sleep
    c. A bedridden client requires more frequent back rubs because of the potential for skin breakdown
2. Purpose
    a. To encourage relaxation
    b. To relieve muscle tension
    c. To stimulate circulation to tissues and muscles
    d. To assess the client's skin
3. Procedure
    a. Help the client to the edge of the bed and into a prone or sidelying position
    b. Expose the back, shoulders, and buttocks; cover the rest of the client's body with a bath blanket
    c. Place a towel alongside the client's back
    d. Wash and warm your hands in warm water
    e. Warm lotion, and pour a small amount into the palms
    f. Place hands on the client's back, and rub in a circular motion over the sacral areas
    g. Stroke upward, along the center of the back, from buttocks to shoulders
    h. Massage in a circular motion over the scapulae
    i. Move hands along the side of the back down to the iliac crests; massage areas over the right and left iliac crests
    j. Repeat strokes for 3 to 5 minutes
    k. Inspect skin for possible breakdown
    l. Wipe lotion from the client's back with a bath towel
    m. Wash hands

4. Documentation
   a. Document the back rub on the flowsheet or in the nurses' notes
   b. Record the client's skin condition and any redness or broken areas
5. Nursing considerations
   a. Assess the condition of the client's skin during the back rub
   b. Offer a back rub to a client after a bath or when the client prepares for sleep
   c. Never rub the lower legs, especially the calves, to prevent movement of possible blood clot
   d. Avoid using alcohol for back rubs because of its drying effect

F. Bedmaking

1. General information
   a. Bed linen is changed for aseptic and comfort reasons
   b. Beds are made after a complete or partial bed bath because the bed may become wet or soiled during the bath
   c. Used linens harbor microorganisms that can be transmitted to others directly or indirectly by the nurse's hands or uniform
   d. Soiled linen is placed directly in a laundry bag or portable hamper; it is never shaken in the air
   e. Types of bedmaking include *unoccupied* (bed is made when the client is sitting in a chair or ambulating), *occupied* (bed is made when the client is in bed, unable to get out even for short periods), and *surgical* or *postoperative* (bed is made for a client undergoing surgery that requires anesthesia)
2. Purpose
   a. To provide a clean environment
   b. To promote client comfort
   c. To reduce transmission of microorganisms
3. Procedure: Making an unoccupied bed
   a. Gather and arrange supplies: laundry bag, two flat sheets, drawsheet (optional in some institutions), blanket, bedspread, waterproof pad (optional), and pillowcases on bedside table or chair
   b. Wash hands
   c. Lower siderails and adjust bed to working height
   d. Loosen all linens while moving around the bed; fold linens to be reused in fourths and hang over the bedside chair
   e. Roll soiled linens away from your body and immediately place them into a laundry bag; do not hold linens against uniform or place on the floor or furniture because of the potential spread of pathogens from soiled linens
   f. Slide the mattress to the head of the bed
   g. Place the center fold of the bottom sheet in the middle of the bed; fanfold half of the sheet toward the opposite side of the bed; make sure the hem of the bottom edge is seam side down and even with the bottom of the mattress

HOW TO MITER A CORNER

To miter a corner, first tuck the end of the sheet evenly under the mattress at the head of the bed. Then lift the side edge of the sheet about 12″ (30.5 cm) from the mattress corner (1) and hold it at a right angle to the mattress (2). Next, tuck in the bottom edge of the sheet hanging below the mattress (3). Finally, drop the top edge and tuck it under the mattress (4, 5, and 6).

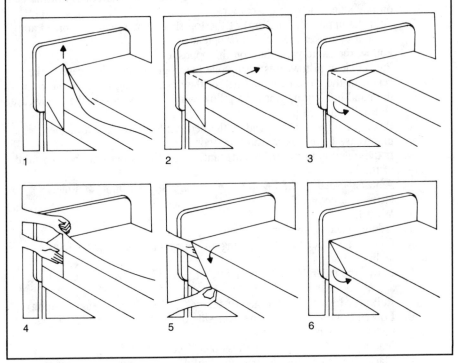

h. Tuck the bottom sheet securely under the head of the mattress, and miter the top corner (see *How to miter a corner*)
i. Tuck the side of the bottom sheet under the mattress
j. Lay the center fold of the drawsheet along the middle of the bed lengthwise so that it will be under the client's chest-to-knee area; if using a waterproof pad, place under the drawsheet
k. Tuck in the side of the drawsheet
l. Move to the opposite side of the bed
m. Starting at the head of the bed, tuck the bottom sheet under the head of the mattress and miter the top corner

    n. Pull the remainder of the sheet tightly, and tuck under the mattress; repeat the same for the drawsheet

    o. Place the center fold of the top sheet in the middle of the bed; place the top of the sheet so that one hem is even with the head of the mattress

    p. Unfold the top sheet in place; then follow the same procedure for the blanket or bedspread

    q. Tuck the top sheet and blanket or bedspread under the bottom of the bed on one side, mitering the corner

    r. Fold the upper 6" (15.2 cm) of the top sheet down over the spread and make a cuff over the blanket or spread

    s. Follow the same procedure on the opposite side

    t. Put on clean pillowcases: using one hand, grasp the pillowcase at the center of the closed end and gather the case, turning it inside out over the hand holding it; grasp the pillow with the hand inside the pillowcase and pull onto the pillow

    u. Place the pillow at the head of the bed, with the open end of the pillowcase facing away from the door

    v. If the client is to return to bed, fanfold top linens onto the bottom third of the bed

    w. Adjust the bed to the low position, secure the call light, and help the client into bed

    x. Wash hands

4. Procedure: Making an occupied bed

    a. Follow the procedure for making an unoccupied bed, with a few additional steps

    b. Lower the siderail on the near side of the bed, leaving the opposite siderail up

    c. Roll the client to the far side of the bed and into a sidelying position

    d. Loosen bottom linens on the near side of the bed; tuck soiled linens under the client

    e. Smooth wrinkles on the mattress pad if not changed

    f. Place clean linens on the bed and fanfold as far under the client as possible

    g. Make the bed in the same manner as for an unoccupied bed

    h. Raise the siderail on the near side, and roll the client over the soiled and clean linens toward the near side

    i. Move to the opposite side, remove soiled linens, and complete making the bed

    j. Secure the top linen as for making an unoccupied bed

5. Procedure: Making a surgical bed

    a. Follow the procedure for making an unoccupied bed, except for the top linens

    b. Place top linens on the bed but do not tuck in

    c. Fold top linens one quarter down from the top and bottom

    d. Fanfold linens to the side opposite from the one the client will enter

    e. Leave the bed in a high position to facilitate client transfer from stretcher to bed

    f. Change pillowcases as suggested for making an unoccupied bed but leave pillows on the bedside chair

6. Documentation

    a. Bedmaking is not usually documented

    b. Be sure to document unusual circumstances, such as drainage or blood observed on sheets

7. Nursing considerations

    a. Remove any personal items or equipment from bedding before changing sheets so that these articles are not discarded with the linens

    b. Determine the client's condition and tolerance for being out of bed

    c. Assess the amount of movement and type of position the client can safely assume during the making of an occupied bed

    d. Maintain proper body alignment when moving and positioning the client

    e. Move the client safely, gently, smoothly, and appropriately for his condition

    f. Work on one side of the bed at a time to minimize client position changes

    g. Enlist the help of a second nurse if the client is weak or debilitated

    h. When making an occupied bed, organize equipment to minimize client position changes

Points to Remember

Factors influencing hygienic practices include the client's culture, socioeconomic status, religion, developmental level, health status, and personal preference.

A nurse assists the client in meeting hygiene needs by providing care that the client alone cannot or should not provide.

A complete bed bath consists of washing a dependent client's entire body in bed.

During the bath, the nurse assesses the client's skin for rash, redness, dryness, or breakdown.

Frequency of mouth care depends on the condition of the client's mouth and comfort.

Occupied bedmaking should be organized to minimize client position changes.

Glossary

Emollient — substance that softens tissues, especially skin

Miter — process of folding and tucking the corner of a bed sheet to prevent it from loosening easily

Sordes — debris that accumulates in the mouth during illness

Promoting Safety and Mobility

Learning Objectives

After studying this section, the reader should be able to:

- Discuss the use of body mechanics in moving, transferring, and ambulating clients.

- Describe how clients should be moved, transferred, and ambulated.

- Cite the purpose of range-of-motion exercises.

- Describe nursing responsibilities when using restraints.

- Discuss the care of a client with a recently applied cast.

V. Promoting Safety and Mobility

A. Introduction

1. Mobility refers to a person's ability to move about
   a. When a client becomes immobile (unable to move), each body system is at risk for dysfunction
   b. Alterations in mobility can be temporary or permanent, minimal or extensive
2. Nursing procedures are directed toward restoring optimal mobility and preventing some of the effects of immobility
   a. Immobility can decrease lung expansion and muscle mass and cause pressure ulcer formation, stasis of urine, renal calculus formation, kidney infection, fecal impaction, behavioral changes, depression, and changes in the sleep-awake cycle
   b. Nursing procedures related to client mobility include moving, transferring, ambulating, frequent repositioning, and range-of-motion exercises
3. When performing these procedures, a nurse uses correct body mechanics—the efficient use of body weight, coordination, and strength
4. Proper alignment of both the nurse's and client's body reduces the probability of injury
5. A client with altered mobility must receive some type of exercise to prevent excessive muscle atrophy and joint contracture and to maintain muscle and joint function

B. Positioning, moving, and transferring a client

1. General information
   a. Correct positioning, moving, and transferring of a client maintains body alignment, prevents injury, and deters pressure ulcer formation
   b. Before moving or transferring a client, the nurse assesses the client's ability to assist, determines the safest method to use, and evaluates how much assistance is required
   c. Whenever a client's health permits, the nurse encourages client involvement
   d. Body mechanics techniques are used to protect the client and nurse from injury (see *Using body mechanics*)
   e. Clients are commonly placed in various positions, including Fowler's (on the back, with the head of the bed elevated 60 to 90 degrees), semi-Fowler's (on the back, with the head of the bed elevated 30 to 45 degrees), supine (on the back, with the head of the bed flat), lateral (sidelying), Sims' (sidelying, with upper leg flexed), and prone (lying face down)
   f. To position a client in proper alignment, a nurse can use positioning aids, such as pillows, trochanter roll, footboard, bedboard, siderails, trapeze bar, and bed cradles

---

USING BODY MECHANICS

● Before lifting, moving, or transferring a client, "put on" the internal girdle by contracting the gluteal muscles in the buttocks downward and the abdominal muscles upward.
● Begin lifting, moving, and transferring activities by broadening the base of support and lowering the center of gravity. Place the feet apart to provide a wide base of support when needed.
● Flex the knees and use the body's

weight to push or pull the object, using a rocking motion.
● Work as closely as possible to the object being lifted or moved.
● Slide, roll, push, or pull an object rather than lift it to reduce the energy needed to move the weight against the pull of gravity.
● Use the longest and strongest muscles of the arms and legs, not the back muscles.

---

    g. When moving a client, a nurse can use a draw sheet (also called a pull or turning sheet), a transfer board, a mechanical lift (such as a Hoyer lift), and smooth dry foundation sheets to help decrease friction, which increases the effort required to move an object

2. Purpose
    a. To reduce hazards of immobility
    b. To promote proper body alignment
    c. To promote the client's comfort
3. Procedure: Helping a supine client move to the head of the bed
    a. Place the head of the bed flat
    b. Fold the client's arms across the chest, or instruct the client to grasp a trapeze bar
    c. Stand next to and face the head of the bed, with feet apart, one foot slightly in front of the other, and knees bent
    d. Ask the client to bend the knees and place the feet flat on the bed, or, if unable to move the legs, to hold onto siderails
    e. Place one hand and arm under the client's shoulder and the other hand under the thighs
    f. Rock backward then forward, pushing the client's body upward while the client pushes off with the legs or arms
4. Procedure: Moving a client up in bed with a draw sheet (two nurses)
    a. Fold a sheet in half, and place it across the bed under the client from shoulder to thighs
    b. Gather or roll each side of the draw sheet close to the client's body
    c. Grasp each side of the pull sheet near the client's shoulder and hip
    d. Tell the client to push off with the legs or arms, as both nurses lift and pull the sheet and the client's body in the same direction
5. Procedure: Moving a client by logrolling (three nurses)
    a. Ask another nurse to stand with you on one side of the client's bed, and ask a third nurse to stand at the head of the bed
    b. Cross the client's arms on the chest

    c. Place your arms under the client's neck and thoracic spine, and have the second nurse place her arms under the client's lumbar spine and knees; for a client with a cervical neck injury, the third nurse should maintain alignment of the client's head and neck

    d. Pull the client to the side of the bed

    e. Place a pillow lengthwise between the client's knees and thighs, and place a small pillow where it will support the client's head after the turn

    f. Move to the opposite side of the bed; with the other nurses, roll the client at the same time so that the body moves as a unit into the lateral position

6. Procedure: Transferring a client from a bed to a chair

    a. Move the prone client to the side of the bed into a high Fowler's position

    b. Place a chair next to and facing the head of the bed

    c. Help the client into a dangling position: place the arm nearer to the head of the bed under the client's shoulder and support the head and neck, and place the other arm over the client's thighs; move the legs and feet over the side of the bed and allow the client's lower legs to swing downward while moving the torso into a sitting position; lower the bed until the client's feet touch the floor

    d. Continue supporting the client in a sitting position, and wait several seconds to determine whether the client is dizzy or lightheaded

    e. Bend your knees and hips so that your upper body is at the same level as the client's upper body; use a wide stance with one foot forward

    f. Tell the client to place arms and hands on your shoulders; then place your hands on the client's ribs, just above waist level

    g. Ask the client to rise slowly to a standing position; place your front knee against the client's opposite knee; raise and support the arising client

    h. Help the client turn until the back is next to the chair seat; instruct the client to sit down when the back of the legs touches the edge of the seat; hold the client under the axillae until sitting is completed

7. Procedure: Transferring a client from a bed to a stretcher (two or three nurses)

    a. Lower the head of the bed flat, and lock the wheels

    b. Raise the bed slightly higher than the stretcher

    c. Pull the draw sheet out from both sides of the bed; roll edges as close as possible to the client's sides

    d. Pull the client to the edge of the bed where the stretcher will be positioned

    e. Place the stretcher parallel to the bed, and lock the wheels

    f. Press your body tightly against the stretcher toward the bed, roll the drawsheet tightly against the client, and, in one motion, pull the client onto the stretcher

    g. Raise the stretcher's siderails, and fasten safety straps across the client

8. Procedure: Assisting a client with ambulation

    a. Plan the length of the walk and rest points with the client

    b. Place the bed in a low position, and help the client to sit upright; then let the client sit or stand for a few minutes to gain balance

    c. Stand behind the client; place both hands at the client's waist or use a walking belt to provide support

    d. If the client has weakness on one side, provide added support by standing on that side; place an arm around the client's waist and the client's arm around your shoulder

    e. Step forward, using the leg opposite to that used by the client

    f. Walk for the time and distance planned, stopping at designated rest points

    g. If the client starts to fall, try to lean the client's body backward so that your body provides support; then gently lower the client to the floor and call for assistance

9. Documentation

    a. Note any position changes or special methods used, such as logrolling a client with a neck injury

    b. Document when a client sits in a chair or ambulates, the activity's duration, and (for ambulation) the distance covered

    c. Record the client's response to position changes, sitting in a chair, and ambulation

10. Nursing considerations

    a. Assess the client's need for help and ability to assist with moving, position changes, transferring, and ambulation

    b. Anticipate the need for additional nurses so that the client is not kept waiting or time is not lost while assistance is obtained

    c. Follow principles of body mechanics

    d. Use aids, such as a draw sheet, transfer board, or mechanical lift

    e. Protect the client's privacy at all times

    f. Maintain safety by using siderails, positioning aids, and transfer devices when appropriate

    g. Place the client's arms across the chest or next to the body before any move to prevent injury

    h. Lower the siderail only on the side of the bed where a nurse is standing and assisting the client

    i. Lock wheels of a bed, wheelchair, or stretcher before transferring a client

    j. Assess the client's position after a move, and maintain correct body alignment

    k. Check vital signs if the client complains of dizziness when moving from one position to another

C. Range-of-motion exercises

1. General information

    a. Full range of motion (ROM) refers to the maximum movement possible for a joint

    b. ROM exercises are performed three to four times daily to maintain joint function (see *Range-of-motion exercises,* pages 53 to 55)

    c. *Active* ROM exercises are performed by the client with supervision and encouragement from a nurse; they have the added benefit of increasing muscle tone

    d. *Active-assistive* exercises are performed by the client, who moves the joints as far as possible, and a nurse or physical therapist, who moves the joints up to the normal range

    e. *Passive* exercises are performed by a nurse or physical therapist for a client who cannot perform them

    f. *Isometric* exercises do not maintain joint mobility but help preserve muscle strength and tone

2. Purpose

    a. To maintain muscle tone and strength and prevent muscle atrophy

    b. To cause muscles to contract; to maintain size, shape, and strength of muscles; to maintain joint mobility (active)

    c. To encourage normal muscle function (active-assistive)

    d. To maintain joint mobility and to prevent contractures and joint stiffness (passive)

3. Procedure: Performing active ROM exercises

    a. Determine where the client will perform the exercises—in bed, sitting, or standing

    b. Teach active ROM exercises through demonstration or use of visual aids

    c. Tell the client that each joint should be put through its range three to five times

    d. Observe the client performing the exercises

4. Procedure: Performing passive ROM exercises

    a. Explain the purpose of the procedure to the client

    b. Position the client supine, with the bed as flat as possible

    c. Expose only the limb being exercised

    d. Provide support above and below the joint, using a cradling or cupping action

    e. Use a firm, comfortable grip when handling the limb

    f. Move the body parts smoothly, slowly, and rhythmically

5. Documentation

    a. Document the frequency with which the client performs the exercises

    b. Record the client's response, including any pain or discomfort

    c. Note any changes in joint condition or mobility

6. Nursing considerations

    a. Be aware that joint swelling and inflammation may contraindicate ROM exercises; report such findings to the charge nurse or physician

    b. Explain to the client that each joint will be bent, straightened, or rotated in a slow, smooth, and rhythmic fashion at least three times

    c. To avoid injury, do not force a body part beyond the existing range of motion

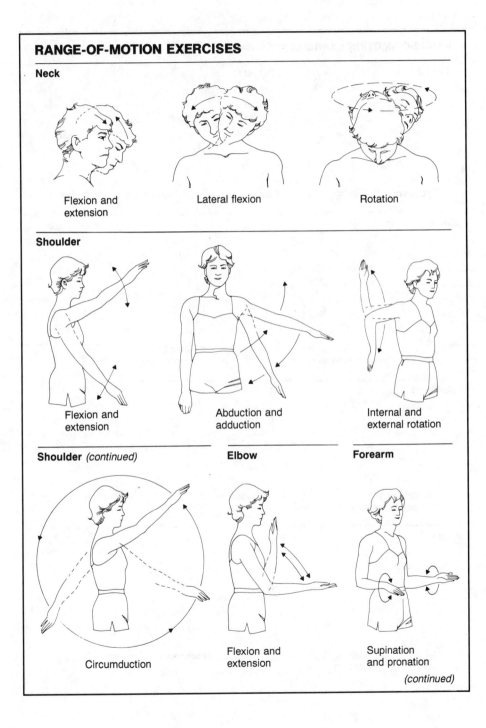

RANGE-OF-MOTION EXERCISES

Neck

Flexion and extension

Lateral flexion

Rotation

Shoulder

Flexion and extension

Abduction and adduction

Internal and external rotation

Shoulder *(continued)*

Elbow

Forearm

Circumduction

Flexion and extension

Supination and pronation

(continued)

RANGE-OF-MOTION EXERCISES *(continued)*

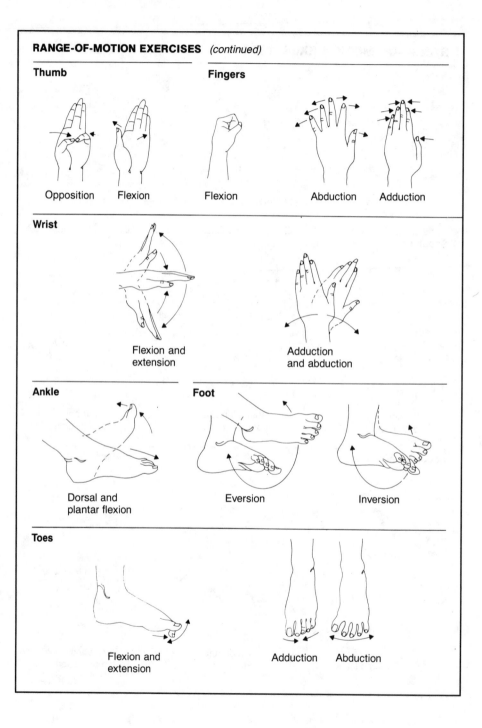

Thumb

Opposition   Flexion

Fingers

Flexion   Abduction   Adduction

Wrist

Flexion and
extension

Adduction
and abduction

Ankle

Dorsal and
plantar flexion

Foot

Eversion   Inversion

Toes

Flexion and
extension

Adduction   Abduction

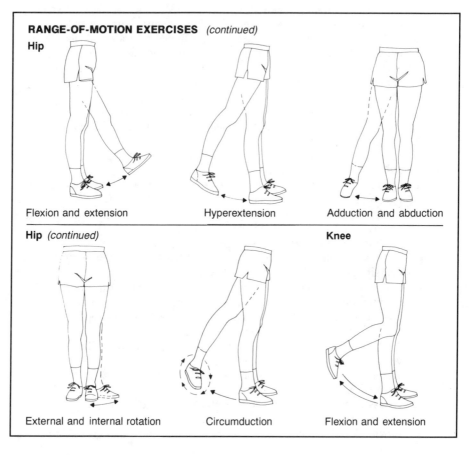

RANGE-OF-MOTION EXERCISES *(continued)*

Hip

Flexion and extension   Hyperextension   Adduction and abduction

Hip *(continued)*   **Knee**

External and internal rotation   Circumduction   Flexion and extension

D. Restraint application

1. General information

   a. Restraints are devices used to limit a client's movements

   b. A physician's order is required to apply restraints, unless the client risks self-harm or is a danger to others

   c. The nurse must know what type of restraint to use — jacket, extremity (ankle or wrist), mitten, elbow, mummy, or belt — and when a restraint is necessary

   d. A *jacket restraint* is a vestlike garment that usually crosses in back of the client

   e. An *extremity restraint* immobilizes one or all extremities and is usually made of sheepskin, foam, cotton, or leather

   f. A thumbless *mitten restraint* immobilizes the client's hands and is usually made of cotton, mesh, or gauze

  g. An *elbow restraint* is made of cotton or muslin and has slots in which tongue blades are placed so that the elbow joint remains extended

  h. A *mummy restraint* is a blanket or sheet folded over a client, usually a child, to ensure security during a procedure, such as intravenous line insertion

  i. A *belt restraint* secures the client on the stretcher

2. Purpose

  a. To prevent the client from falling out of a bed, stretcher, or chair

  b. To avoid interruption of therapy, such as intravenous infusions or nasogastric tube feedings

  c. To reduce the risk of self-inflicted injury or injury to others

3. Procedure: Applying restraints

  a. Obtain a physician's order for a restraint that limits a client's motion or immobilizes him

  b. Explain to the client and family members why a restraint is needed, the type selected, and the expected duration of use

  c. Assemble equipment, including the proper restraint

  d. Pad bony prominences, such as wrists and ankles, before putting the restraint over them

  e. Follow the manufacturer's directions, and allow the greatest degree of mobility possible without defeating the purpose of the restraint

  f. Place body parts in their normal anatomic position, and apply the restraint to the body area specified in the physician's order

  g. Tie the restraint with a knot, such as a clove hitch, that will not tighten when pulled

  h. Fasten the restraint to parts of the bedframe that move when the bed is elevated; never attach a restraint to siderails

  i. Assess circulation of the restrained body part after 30 minutes; loosen and remove the restraint at least every 2 hours

  j. Provide ROM exercises to the restrained body part, and give skin care as indicated

4. Documentation

  a. Record nursing measures employed to avoid use of restraints

  b. Document client behavior that led to restraints

  c. Note the type of restraint used, time applied and removed, assessment of circulation, and loosening of restraint

  d. Document client behavior while the restraint is in place

  e. Log any notification of the physician

  f. Document the explanation given to the client and family members for use of restraints

5. Nursing considerations

  a. Explain to the client and family that restraints are protective devices, not punishment

  b. Know the institution's policy and practices and the state laws governing client restraint

    c. Try other nursing measures (such as talking with the client, raising siderails, or administering a prescribed sedative) before applying restraints

    d. Be aware that restraints can cause injury or skin irritation and impair blood flow if applied incorrectly

    e. Use restraints only to ensure the safety of the client or others

    f. Choose the restraint that best meets the client's needs

E. Cast care

  1. General information

    a. A cast is a rigid dressing or bandage that immobilizes an injured limb or other body part to prevent further damage and permit healing

    b. It is applied by wrapping long, moistened bandages around the limb; the bandages harden as they dry, forming a rigid mold

    c. Plaster of Paris casts take 24 to 48 hours to dry; the cast may crack or break if not protected while drying

  2. Purpose

    a. To protect the client from effects of constricted circulation after the cast is applied

    b. To protect the cast from damage

  3. Procedure: Caring for a client with a recently applied cast

    a. Handle the cast with palms, not fingers

    b. Place the limb with the cast on pillows to encourage venous return and prevent swelling

    c. Turn the limb every 2 hours to promote uniform drying

    d. Regularly assess the neurovascular status of the extremity distal to the cast

  4. Documentation

    a. Record neurovascular assessment of the extremity distal to the cast, including color, pulses, and sensation

    b. Note the cast's condition and nursing measures used to facilitate drying

    c. Document the client's response, including discomfort and pain

  5. Nursing considerations

    a. Tell the client not to slip any object under the cast; if an object does become stuck, inform the physician

    b. Notify the physician of any change in neurovascular status, such as swelling, loss of sensation, absence of pulse, or change of color

    c. After the cast dries, petal the edges to prevent skin irritation

    d. Cover cast edges near the perineal area with plastic, rubber, oiled cloth, or waxed paper to protect the cast from urine and feces

    e. Avoid covering the entire cast with waterproof material for prolonged periods because the cast cannot "breathe" and may cause skin maceration (the cast can be covered for a short time during bathing)

Points to Remember

Techniques of body mechanics are used to protect the client and nurse from injury.

Before moving, transferring, or ambulating a client, the nurse determines the client's ability to assist in the procedure, the safest method to use, and how much assistance is required.

ROM exercises are performed three to four times daily to maintain joint function.

A physician's order is required to apply restraints.

Restraints are potentially hazardous to the client.

The nurse should regularly assess the client's circulation in the body part distal to where a restraint or cast has been applied.

Glossary

Alignment — proper positioning of body parts along a straight line

Contracture — abnormal and usually permanent condition of a joint caused by atrophy and shortening of muscle fibers

Isometric exercises — exercises that strengthen and increase muscle tone by forcing the muscles to contract against resistance (from other muscles or from a stationary object, such as a bed or wall)

Neurovascular assessment — evaluation of the nervous system and circulation in a body part constricted by a cast, bandage, or restraint; includes assessment of capillary refill, edema, color, temperature, movement, and sensation

Petal — to place strips of adhesive or moleskin over a cast's edges to prevent them from rubbing against the skin and causing irritation

Walking belt — a leather device that supports a client's waist during ambulation; the device has handles for a nurse to hold

Ensuring Urinary Elimination

Learning Objectives

After studying this section, the reader should be able to:

● List five nursing measures for assisting a client to void.

● Describe the procedure for measuring fluid intake and output.

● Cite the purpose of urinary catheterization.

● Review nursing care of a client before and after catheterization.

● Explain the procedure for obtaining a urine specimen from a retention catheter.

VI. Ensuring Urinary Elimination

A. Introduction

1. Elimination of urine is a basic need that removes liquid wastes from the body
   a. Emptying the bladder of urine is called voiding, micturition, or urination
   b. Urine collects in the bladder until pressure stimulates sensory nerve endings that signal the need to urinate
   c. The need to urinate occurs in an adult when the bladder contains 250 to 450 ml of urine and in a child when it contains 50 to 200 ml
   d. Incontinence is the involuntary emptying of the bladder and can be caused by such disorders as brain or spinal cord injury, which results in loss of voluntary control of voiding
   e. Retention is the accumulation of urine in the bladder caused by the inability to urinate
   f. Retention with overflow occurs when a small amount of urine is voided frequently or urine dribbles while the bladder remains distended
2. Altered patterns of voiding include:
   a. Frequency (more often than usual)
   b. Nocturia (increased frequency at night)
   c. Urgency (need to void immediately)
   d. Dysuria (painful or difficult voiding)
   e. Polyuria or diuresis (abnormally large amounts of urine produced)
3. Independent nursing actions to promote urinary elimination include:
   a. Encouraging fluid intake
   b. Providing a relaxed, private setting and a normal position (standing for male, sitting for female)
   c. Running tap water within range of the client's hearing
   d. Pouring water over the client's perineal area or hands
4. Interdependent and dependent nursing actions to promote urinary elimination include:
   a. Measuring fluid intake and output (may also be initiated by the nurse)
   b. Obtaining urine specimens for culture and sensitivity
   c. Inserting a catheter
5. Surgical asepsis is required for a procedure involving the bladder because urine within the bladder is sterile; medical asepsis is required for a procedure involving the urinary meatus, which can be cleaned but is not sterile

B. Fluid intake and output monitoring

1. General information
   a. The term *fluid intake and output* refers to the measurement of all fluids that enter and exit the body
   b. Daily fluid intake and daily fluid output are usually about the same amount

   c. An imbalance (when fluid intake and output are not equal) may indicate
       an unusual or abnormal process, which occurs with certain medications
       (diuretics), kidney diseases, or heart failure
   d. *Intake* includes all food and fluids that are liquid at room temperature
       (such as ice cream and gelatin), parenteral fluids (such as I.V. solutions),
       and any other fluids taken into the body (such as those through tubes)
   e. *Output* includes urine, vomitus, diarrhea, and drainage from suctioning
       devices
   f. Intake and output are gauged using measuring containers whenever
       possible; output may need to be estimated in some situations (for
       example, diarrhea or urine in a diaper or bedclothes)
   g. Each institution has an intake and output (I&O) sheet that the nurse uses
       to record each intake (such as I.V. or oral) or output (such as urine or
       vomitus); a chart giving the volume amounts of commonly used drinking
       containers, such as a coffee cup or soup bowl, usually accompanies the
       I&O sheet
   h. The I&O sheet, usually kept at the bedside for easy recording, is totaled
       every 8 hours (end of each nursing shift) and retotaled every 24 hours
       (usually at the end of the night shift)
2. Purpose
   a. To monitor the client's fluid intake and output
   b. To monitor renal function
3. Procedure: Measuring fluid intake and output
   a. Gather equipment: I&O sheet, pencil, disposable measuring cup or
       graduated bedpan or urinal, and measuring "hat," which is placed under
       the toilet seat for ambulatory clients
   b. Indicate on the nursing care plan that the client is on I&O orders, and
       post a sign stating "intake and output" on his room door or near the bed
   c. Keep the I&O sheet in the client's room
   d. Explain to the client or family members that a record is being kept of
       fluid intake and output, and explain that they can participate by
       monitoring these when the nurse is not in the room
   e. Monitor, measure, and record all fluids that enter the client's body,
       including I.V. and feeding tube fluids, blood, and oral fluids during and
       between meals
   f. Monitor, measure, and record all fluids that leave the client's body,
       including urine from an indwelling catheter, fluids from a nasogastric
       tube, wound drains, vomitus, and liquid stool
4. Documentation
   a. Total the amount of fluid intake and output every 8 hours, and add the
       totals every 24 hours
   b. Document any imbalance or abnormal amount of output in the nurses'
       notes
5. Nursing considerations
   a. Wear clean disposable gloves when measuring urine
   b. Report any abnormal output to the charge nurse or physician

c. For seriously ill catheterized clients, measure urine hourly, using a urinometer; after assessing the hourly amount, empty the urine in the measuring chamber into the general collection bag

C. Urine specimen collection
1. General information
   a. A *clean catch* urine specimen is collected during midstream urination; the first and last parts of the voiding are not collected
   b. The initial voiding helps flush away microorganisms that may be near the meatus; discarding the last part prevents microorganisms that may be retained in the bladder from being introduced into the specimen
   c. A clean catch specimen from a male is sterile; a female must be catheterized if a sterile specimen is needed
   d. The nurse provides the equipment and tells the client how to collect the specimen (or assists in collection, if necessary)
2. Purpose: to obtain a urine specimen that is free from contaminants, especially bacteria
3. Procedure: Obtaining a urine specimen (female)
   a. Gather supplies: clean disposable gloves, sterile container, label, antiseptic solution or soap, plastic bag, washcloth, towel, and warm water (to clean the perineum if it has been contaminated with vaginal secretions or feces)
   b. Wash hands and put on gloves
   c. Open the sterile container and place the lid topside down
   d. Spread the labia, keeping them apart until the specimen is obtained
   e. Clean around the external meatus with antiseptic solution and gauze or cotton balls; move the cotton balls from the meatus toward the anus, using one cotton ball for each stroke (institution policy may require rinsing with sterile water and drying with sterile gauze)
   f. Have the client void about 30 ml into the bedpan or toilet
   g. Position the sterile container near to but not touching the meatus, and collect urine in the container
   h. Tell the client to continue voiding into the bedpan or toilet until the bladder is emptied
   i. Cap the sterile container without touching the inside of the lid, and clean the outside of the container with soap and water
   j. Label the container, place it inside a clean bag, and send it to the laboratory as soon as possible
   k. Dispose of soiled equipment, remove gloves, and wash hands
4. Procedure: Obtaining a urine specimen (male)
   a. Follow the same steps as for obtaining a urine specimen from a female, except for spreading the labia and cleaning the meatus
   b. Clean the area around the meatus using a circular motion, starting at the penis tip and moving down the shaft for several inches
5. Documentation
   a. Record the time and method used to collect the specimen

    b. Note the amount and characteristics of urine

    c. Complete the laboratory slip and document the time the specimen is sent to the laboratory

6. Nursing considerations

    a. Ensure that the specimen label and laboratory requisition form are filled out correctly

    b. Securely attach the label to the container

    c. Send the specimen to the laboratory at once so that bacterial cultures are started before contaminating microorganisms can multiply

    d. Use aseptic technique to keep specimens as free as possible from external contamination by microorganisms near the external meatus

D. Urinary catheterization

1. General information

    a. Urinary catheterization is a procedure in which a tube (catheter) is introduced through the urethra into the bladder

    b. The catheter removes urine in a patient with obstructed flow or retained urine

    c. Catheterization increases the risk of urinary tract infection because bacteria can enter the bladder when the catheter is inserted, and pathogens can move up the tube while the catheter is in place

    d. Catheterization is the most common cause of nosocomial (hospital-acquired) infection and should be avoided when possible; if unavoidable, use sterile technique

2. Urinary catheters

    a. These catheters are made of rubber or plastic and come in many sizes; the higher the number, the larger the catheter (for example, a #22 French catheter is larger than a #16 French catheter)

    b. Indwelling urinary catheters (also called retention or Foley catheters) remain in place for continuous drainage

    c. Intermittent catheters (also called straight catheters) drain the bladder for short periods (5 to 10 minutes)

    d. A suprapubic catheter (used for continuous drainage) is inserted surgically via a small incision above the symphysis pubis

3. Purpose

    a. To relieve urine retention in the bladder

    b. To obtain a sterile urine specimen

    c. To measure residual urine

    d. To maintain bladder decompression during surgery

    e. To monitor hourly urine production

    f. To provide a route for medication instillation or bladder irrigation

    g. To relieve problems associated with incontinence

4. Procedure: Performing indwelling urinary catheterization (in a female client)

    a. Explain catheterization to the client

   b. Assemble equipment: disposable sterile urinary catheterization set, sterile gloves, cotton balls, cleaning solution, specimen container, lubricant, clean disposable gloves, bath blanket, gooseneck lamp or flashlight, catheter of the correct size and type, and appropriate drainage system

   c. Wash hands

   d. Place the client in a dorsal recumbent position, with knees flexed and thighs externally rotated; obtain assistance if the client cannot maintain the required position

   e. Drape the client by placing one corner of the bath blanket around each foot and the other corner over the perineum

   f. Don clean disposable gloves, and wash the perineal area with soap and warm water; then rinse and dry

   g. Adjust the lamp to illuminate the urinary meatus (or have an assistant hold a flashlight)

   h. Open the catheterization set and establish a sterile field; if the set is in a plastic bag, place the bag on the bedside table and use it for waste disposal

   i. Don sterile gloves

   j. Organize supplies on the sterile field: pour antiseptic over cotton balls, lubricate the catheter, check inflation of the catheter balloon with syringe filled with normal saline solution or sterile water, and remove the specimen container from the collection tray compartment

   k. Apply a sterile drape: pick up the underdrape, covering your hands with the corners to protect sterile gloves from touching nonsterile surfaces, and place it under the client's buttocks

   l. Place the sterile tray and contents on the sterile drape between the client's thighs

   m. Clean the urethral meatus: separate labia with thumb and forefinger of the nondominant hand, exposing the meatus (this hand is now contaminated); keep labia separated throughout the procedure; pick up cotton balls with sterile forceps; clean the urinary meatus and surrounding tissue from the clitoris to the anus, using a new cotton ball for each stroke

   n. Pick up the catheter 2″ to 3″ (5 to 8 cm) from the insertion tip with the gloved, uncontaminated hand

   o. Place the catheter's distal end in the urine collection tray and gently insert the catheter tip; when urine appears, advance the catheter another 2″

   p. Leave the catheter in place if inserted into the vagina by mistake, and place a second sterile catheter into the urethra; then remove the first catheter

   q. Release the labia when urine flows, and hold the catheter in place; inflate the balloon with the syringe and sterile water provided in the catheterization set

   r. If the client complains of sudden pain, aspirate the solution and advance the catheter

    s. Attach one end of the catheter to the drainage system tubing; attach the drainage bag to the bed, at a level below the bladder

    t. Wipe the perineum with the drape and remove gloves

    u. Anchor the catheter with tape to the inside of the client's thigh

    v. Coil excess tubing and fasten it to the bed with tape, a tubing clamp, or a rubber band and safety pin; ensure that tubing is not kinked or obstructed

    w. Dispose of all equipment and wash hands

5. Procedure: Performing indwelling urinary catheterization (in a male client)

    a. Follow the same procedure as for indwelling urinary catheterization of a female client, except for positioning, draping, and cleaning

    b. Place the client in a supine position, with hip joints slightly abducted

    c. Apply a sterile drape over the client's thighs, near the penis, and place a second fenestrated drape over the penis and pubic area, exposing only the penis

    d. Clean the area: elevate the penis 60 to 90 degrees and retract the foreskin, if present, with the nondominant hand (now contaminated); clean the meatus first, using cotton balls held by sterile forceps; wipe the surrounding area in a circular motion; discard each cotton ball after use

    e. Pick up the catheter 3″ to 4″ (8 to 10 cm) from the insertion tip with the gloved, uncontaminated hand

    f. Insert the catheter gently until urine appears; lift the penis perpendicular to the body and apply light traction; if slight resistance is felt at the sphincters, rotate the catheter and ask the client to take deep breaths; discontinue if resistance continues and call the physician

    g. When urine flows, lower the penis and inflate the catheter balloon, continuing the procedure as described for a female client

    h. Anchor the catheter to the top of the thigh or to the lower abdomen

6. Procedure: Performing intermittent catheterization

    a. Follow the same procedure as for indwelling urinary catheterization, with a few exceptions

    b. Before inserting a straight, single-use catheter, place the distal end in the urine collection tray

    c. Insert the catheter until urine flow holds the catheter in place

    d. Obtain a urine specimen, if ordered: pinch the catheter, allow urine to flow into the collection bottle, cover the bottle, and set aside to label and send to the laboratory

    e. Allow the client's bladder to empty completely, or limit the amount drained to 700 to 1,000 ml, as specified by institution policy

    f. Remove the catheter by pinching the tubing and withdrawing the catheter slowly

7. Documentation

    a. Document the reason for catheterization (such as bladder distention or preparation for surgery) and the time performed

    b. Record the amount, color, clarity, and odor of urine

      c. Note the type and size of the catheter used and the amount of fluid used to inflate the balloon

      d. Record when the specimen is sent to the laboratory

  8. Nursing considerations

      a. Use principles of surgical asepsis when catheterizing a client and in daily care of a client with an indwelling catheter to prevent transfer of pathogens through the catheter into the bladder

      b. Before catheterizing a client, check the physician's order and assess the client's need for catheterization

      c. Never force a catheter against resistance; withdraw the catheter and notify the physician

      d. Know that a client may experience dysuria and decreased bladder tone if an indwelling catheter is left in place for more than a few days

      e. Deflate the balloon completely before removing an indwelling catheter to prevent trauma to the urethra and meatus

E. Urine specimen collection (indwelling catheter)

  1. General information

      a. Obtaining a urine specimen from a client who has an indwelling catheter requires strict aseptic technique to prevent introduction of pathogens into the urinary tract

      b. The specimen is not collected from the urine drainage bag unless it is the first urine to drain into a sterile bag

  2. Purpose

      a. To isolate specific bacteria causing a urinary tract infection

      b. To obtain a specimen for other tests

  3. Procedure: Withdrawing a urine specimen from an indwelling catheter

      a. Assemble supplies: syringe with 25G needle, sterile specimen container, antiseptic swabs, rubber band or clamp, and clean disposable gloves

      b. Wash hands

      c. Clamp drainage tubing below the collection port with a rubber band or clamp 5 to 10 minutes before collecting urine

      d. Wash hands and don gloves

      e. Wipe the entry port with an antiseptic swab

      f. Insert the needle at an angle into the entry port, and aspirate 2 to 3 ml of urine for a culture or 20 ml of urine for routine urinalysis

      g. Transfer urine into the prepared specimen container

      h. Cover the container, maintaining sterility inside the lid

      i. Unclamp the catheter tubing

      j. Label the container and send it to the laboratory within 15 minutes; if specified by institution policy, place the specimen inside a plastic bag for transport

      k. Discard soiled equipment, remove gloves, and wash hands

  4. Documentation

      a. Chart the time of urine collection and the amount, color, clarity, and odor of the urine

b. Document the time the specimen was sent to the laboratory
5. Nursing considerations
   a. Use sterile technique when inserting a catheter to prevent contamination by pathogens
   b. Label the urine specimen carefully, and send it to the laboratory within 15 minutes

F. Indwelling catheter removal
1. General information
   a. An indwelling catheter remains in place until the physician writes an order to remove it
   b. The client's bladder may need time to reestablish full voluntary control after the catheter has been withdrawn; involuntary voiding is not unusual
2. Purpose: to reestablish normal voiding
3. Procedure: Removing an indwelling catheter
   a. Assemble equipment: syringe (of the same size as the volume of solution used to inflate the balloon), clean disposable gloves, and waterproof pad
   b. Wash hands and don clean gloves
   c. Place the client in a supine position, and put the waterproof pad between the client's thighs
   d. Obtain a sterile urine specimen if ordered
   e. Remove tape used to secure the catheter
   f. Insert the syringe into the inflation valve, and aspirate the total amount of fluid used to inflate the balloon
   g. Pull the catheter out slowly, using a continuous motion, and wrap the contaminated catheter in the waterproof pad
   h. Measure and empty the contents of the urine collection bag
4. Documentation
   a. Record when the catheter is removed and when the specimen is sent to the laboratory
   b. Note the amount and characteristics of the urine remaining in the collection bag
5. Nursing considerations
   a. After removing the indwelling catheter, monitor intake and output for at least 24 hours and assess the client for signs of urine retention
   b. If the client has not voided within 8 hours after catheter removal, check the physician's order to see if the catheter may be reinserted

G. External catheterization
1. General information
   a. An external catheter, also known as a condom catheter or Texas catheter, is a urinary drainage device placed over the penis that collects urine as it is voided
   b. The external catheter is preferred over an indwelling catheter because it minimizes infection risk

2. Purpose
   a. To collect urine from an incontinent male
   b. To keep bedding and clothing dry, thus reducing the risk of skin breakdown
3. Procedure: Applying an external catheter
   a. Assemble equipment: condom sheath of appropriate size, basin of warm water and soap, bath blanket, clean disposable gloves, washcloth and towel, elastic or Velcro adhesive, reusable leg bag or urine collection bag with drainage tubing
   b. Explain the procedure to the client and provide privacy
   c. Wash hands
   d. Help the client into a supine position, place the bath blanket over the upper body, and cover the legs with a bedsheet, exposing the penis
   e. Don clean gloves
   f. Wash the penis with soap and water, rinse, and dry thoroughly
   g. Roll the condom sheath outward onto itself
   h. Grasp the penis firmly along the shaft with the nondominant hand, and roll the condom sheath smoothly onto the penile shaft with the dominant hand
   i. Leave 1″ to 2″ (2.5 to 5 cm) between the penis tip and the end of the condom
   j. Place an elastic or Velcro strap snugly around the condom at the base of the penis
   k. Connect the condom sheath to drainage tubing
4. Documentation
   a. Record the procedure and the condition of the client's skin
   b. Chart the amount and characteristics of the urine
5. Nursing considerations
   a. Change the condom daily or according to institution policy
   b. Check the foreskin and the shaft of the penis for swelling, discoloration, or irritation within 30 minutes of applying the condom and every 8 hours thereafter
   c. Assess the amount, color, clarity, and odor of urine

H. Catheter irrigation
1. General information
   a. Irrigation is the flushing of a tube, canal, or area with solution
   b. Bladder, or catheter, irrigation is performed to maintain or restore the catheter's patency
   c. *Closed catheter irrigation* provides intermittent or continuous irrigation without disconnecting the catheter from its drainage system; it is used for clients at risk for occlusion of the catheter with blood clots and mucous fragments after genitourinary surgery

   d. *Open catheter irrigation,* an alternate method, requires that the nurse
      aseptically break the closed drainage system; this method is used
      intermittently to maintain catheter patency but should be done only when
      necessary because of the risk of introducing pathogens into the bladder
   e. Medication can be administered with either method to treat infection or
      local bladder irritation
2. Purpose
   a. To restore or maintain catheter patency
   b. To irrigate the catheter continuously when blood clots or other debris
      may block tubing
   c. To infuse medication into the bladder
3. Procedure: Irrigating a catheter (closed method)
   a. Gather supplies: sterile basin, sterile irrigating solution, alcohol swabs,
      waterproof pad, 18G or 19G needle, 30- to 50-ml syringe
   b. Place the waterproof pad under the catheter and aspiration port
   c. Open sterile supplies, and pour the irrigating solution into the basin
   d. Draw the irrigating solution into the syringe, and attach the needle with
      the cap still in place
   e. Wipe the aspiration port with an alcohol swab, using a firm circular
      motion
   f. Clamp or fold tubing distal to the aspiration port, uncap the needle and
      insert it into the port, and gently instill solution into the catheter
   g. Remove the needle and unclamp tubing, allowing the solution and urine
      to drain; repeat as necessary
   h. Dispose of equipment and wash hands
4. Procedure: Irrigating a catheter (open method)
   a. Assemble supplies: sterile irrigating solution, disposable sterile irrigation
      tray (new set for each irrigation), sterile gloves, collection basin,
      waterproof pad, alcohol pads, and a 30- to 50-ml syringe
   b. Wash hands
   c. Open the sterile tray and establish a sterile field, pouring the prescribed
      solution into the sterile basin and preparing the syringe with solution
   d. Don sterile gloves, position the waterproof pad under the end of the
      catheter, and place the collection basin on the pad
   e. Disconnect the catheter from the drainage tube, and cover the open end
      of the tube with a sterile protective cap
   f. Place the catheter over the edge of the collection basin, but do not allow
      the catheter's open end to touch a nonsterile surface
   g. Instill 30 to 50 ml of solution into the bladder; remove the syringe and
      allow the solution to drain into the basin; repeat irrigation until fluid
      runs clear or clots are removed
   h. Wipe the catheter ends and the drainage tube with alcohol pads,
      reconnect the catheter to the tube, and reanchor the catheter with tape
   i. Dispose of contaminated supplies, remove gloves, and wash hands

5. Documentation
   a. Chart the procedure used, the time it was performed, and the type and amount of solution used
   b. Record the amount of solution on an I&O sheet if the client is on I&O orders
   c. Record the client's response to the procedure, including any discomfort
   d. Document catheter patency and urine characteristics before and after irrigation
6. Nursing considerations
   a. Use aseptic technique when irrigating the bladder to prevent infection
   b. Review the physician's order for the type and amount of solution to use and the type of irrigation to perform
   c. Do not force irrigation against resistance; notify the physician

Points to Remember

Independent nursing actions to facilitate urination include encouraging fluid intake, providing privacy, assisting the client to a normal voiding position, running tap water within the client's hearing, and pouring warm water over the perineum.

A clean catch urine specimen is collected midstream; the first and last parts of the voiding are not collected.

Catheterization should be avoided whenever possible because it is the most common cause of nosocomial infections.

Principles of surgical asepsis are used when catheterizing a client or caring for a client with an indwelling catheter to prevent infection.

Glossary

Aspiration — removing fluid from a cavity or tube by applying suction

Distention — swelling of the lower abdomen caused by excessive urine in the bladder

Residual — amount of urine remaining in the bladder after voiding

Retention — accumulation of urine in the bladder caused by the inability to urinate

Urinometer — calibrated measuring chamber built into an indwelling urinary catheter collection bag to measure hourly amounts of urine

Ensuring Gastrointestinal Elimination

Learning Objectives

After studying this section, the reader should be able to:

● List four clinical signs of interference with gastrointestinal elimination.

● Cite the purpose of a nasogastric tube.

● Review the procedure for inserting and irrigating a nasogastric tube and administering an enteral feeding.

● List nursing measures for assisting a client to pass feces.

● Describe the procedure for giving an enema, inserting a rectal tube, and irrigating a colostomy.

VII. Ensuring Gastrointestinal Elimination

A. Introduction

1. Gastrointestinal elimination is a basic need that removes solid waste products from the body, usually through defecation
2. Factors that may hinder normal gastrointestinal elimination include:
   a. Accumulation of flatus (gas), fluids, or feces caused by slowing or stopping of peristalsis
   b. Surgical bypass procedures, such as colostomy
   c. Head or spinal cord injuries
   d. Immobility
   e. Change in diet
   f. Change in usual bowel elimination habits
3. Clinical signs of interference with gastrointestinal elimination include:
   a. Decreased bowel sounds on abdominal auscultation
   b. Distention of the intestines or stomach by flatus
   c. Vomiting
   d. Diarrhea (frequent passage of liquid stool)
   e. Constipation (passage of small, dry, hard stool or no stool)
   f. Fecal impaction (hardened feces in the rectum that cannot be passed, typically accompanied by seepage of liquid stool)
4. Independent nursing measures that promote normal defecation include:
   a. Correctly positioning a client on the toilet or bedpan (thigh flexion increases pressure within the abdomen, and sitting increases downward pressure on the rectum)
   b. Assisting the client with the bedpan or to the toilet as soon as he feels the urge to defecate
   c. Helping the client select foods that contain bulk (fiber)
   d. Encouraging additional fluid intake
   e. Providing privacy
5. Dependent nursing actions that promote normal defecation include:
   a. Suctioning the stomach via a nasogastric tube
   b. Inserting a rectal tube
   c. Caring for a colostomy
   d. Administering an enema
6. Nursing procedures involving the gastrointestinal tract require medical, not surgical, asepsis because the gastrointestinal tract is not sterile

B. Nasogastric tube insertion

1. General information
   a. A nasogastric (NG) tube is passed through the nose, nasopharynx, and esophagus and into the stomach to instill liquid foods or other substances, such as medications, or to withdraw gastric secretions, fluid, or gas (see *Types of nasogastric tubes,* page 74)

TYPES OF NASOGASTRIC TUBES

TYPE	DESCRIPTION	USE
Levin tube	• Rubber or plastic, single lumen, unvented • Can adhere to gastric mucosa and cause injury or obstruction when suction is used	• Decompression • Lavage • Analysis of gastric contents • Feeding
Ewald tube	• Rubber, large gauge, unvented • Inserted through the client's mouth, usually when lavage is necessary	• Lavage • Analysis of gastric contents
Salem sump	• Clear plastic, double lumen, vented • Prevents adherence to gastric mucosa • Vent must not be obstructed or used for irrigation and must be kept above level of client's stomach to prevent gastric reflux	• Decompression • Lavage
Dubbhoff or Keofeed	• Small bore, flexible • Inserted using a stylet, with minimal trauma • Can be inserted into stomach or duodenum • Obstruction more likely because of small diameter • X-ray used to determine placement	• Feeding

    b. Made of plastic, silicone, or rubber, NG tubes come in various lengths, depending on whether the tube is inserted into the stomach or the intestines; the usual size for an adult is #16 or #18 French

    c. Marked with dark lines to assist in proper placement, an NG tube can be attached to an intermittent gastric suction device, such as a Gomco suction machine

    d. A registered nurse usually inserts an NG tube into the stomach, and then only with a physician's order, whereas a physician usually inserts a tube that must be advanced to the intestines; in some institutions, physicians are responsible for inserting NG tubes in unconscious, confused, or delirious clients, preoperative or postoperative gastric surgery clients, those with gastric hemorrhage or abnormalities of the mouth or esophagus, or those who have undergone surgery in those areas

2. Purpose

    a. To decompress or remove flatus and secretions from the stomach before or after surgery

    b. To prevent distention and vomiting from decreased peristalsis after general anesthesia, handling of the bowel during surgery, or bowel obstruction

    c. To remove or dilute ingested poisons

    d. To obtain a specimen of stomach contents or gastric secretions

    e. To provide liquid feedings to maintain fluid, electrolyte, and nutritional balance in a client unable to take food by mouth

3. Procedure: Inserting an NG tube

    a. Discuss the procedure with the client, including an explanation of how the client can help

    b. Assess the client for presence and activity of bowel sounds in all four quadrants; palpate and percuss the abdomen for distention

    c. Inspect the nostrils for patency; have the client alternately occlude each nostril and breathe

    d. Read the physician's order for the type and size of NG tube required and whether the tube will be attached to suction

    e. Assemble equipment: tube of appropriate size (#12, #14, #16, or #18 French for an adult, #6 or #8 French for a child), water-soluble lubricant, flashlight, tongue blade, stethoscope, towel, emesis basin, 1″ (2.5 cm) wide tape, 20-ml syringe or bulb syringe, glass of water with straw, clamp or plug, suction machine (if used), facial tissues, safety pins, and clean disposable gloves

    f. Help the client into a high Fowler's position

    g. Place a towel or disposable pad across the client's chest; keep tissues and the emesis basin nearby

    h. Wash hands and don gloves

    i. Measure insertion length by placing the tube's tip at the tip of the client's nose and extending it to the tip of the earlobe and then to the xiphoid process of the sternum; mark the tube with a piece of tape

    j. Lubricate the first 4″ to 6″ (10 to 15 cm) of the tube with water-soluble lubricant

    k. Tell the client to hyperextend his neck against the pillow; insert the tube through the nostril with the curved end pointing down

    l. Pass the tube along the floor of the nasal passage and toward the ear on that side; provide tissues if the client's eyes water

    m. If the tube meets resistance, withdraw and relubricate it, and insert it in the other nostril; slight pressure is sometimes needed to pass the tube into the nasopharynx

    n. When the tube reaches the oropharynx, instruct the client to bring his head forward and swallow as the tube passes; advance the tube 1″ to 2″ (2.5 to 5 cm) with each swallow; if permitted, allow the client to sip water

    o. If the client coughs, chokes, or gags, stop passing the tube; have the client take a few breaths and sips of water to calm the gag reflex

    p. If the client continues to gag and cough, pull the tube back slightly; using a tongue blade and flashlight, check the back of the throat for coiling of the tube

    q. If the tube coils, withdraw it until it straightens; when the client relaxes, continue to insert tube until the mark is reached

    r. Evaluate tube placement (see *Checking nasogastric tube placement,* page 76)

CHECKING NASOGASTRIC TUBE PLACEMENT

● Ask the client to talk (if the client cannot talk, the tube may be in the respiratory tract).
● Check the posterior oropharynx for tube coiling.
● Attach a syringe or bulb syringe to the end of the tube.
● Place a stethoscope over the abdomen's left upper quadrant.

● Inject 10 to 20 cc of air, and listen for a rush of air over the stomach.
● Aspirate stomach contents.
● Ask the client to roll to the left side if no gastric contents are aspirated (inability to aspirate gastric contents may indicate that the tube tip is stuck to the stomach wall; changing positions can help dislodge the tube).

---

    s. Clamp or plug the tube or attach it to a suction machine, depending on the physician's order

    t. Tape the tube to the client's nose, using a 4″ (10 cm) piece of tape; place one end of the tape over the nose, split the other end, and wrap split ends around the tube as it leaves the nose; to avoid tissue erosion, do not allow the tube to press against the inside of the nose

    u. Loop a rubber band around the tube end, and attach it to the client's gown with a safety pin (or attach a piece of tape to the tube and pin it to the gown)

4. Documentation

    a. Document the type of NG tube used and the time of insertion

    b. Note the client's tolerance of the procedure

    c. Describe the client's condition after tube insertion, including abdominal distention, presence or absence of bowel sounds, vomiting, or unusual drainage

    d. Record how placement was confirmed

    e. On the intake and output sheet, chart the amount of water ingested during insertion and the amount of drainage

    f. Note the color, amount, and characteristics of drainage if the tube is connected to a suction device

5. Nursing considerations

    a. Obtain assistance if the client is confused or disoriented, and anticipate the need for soft arm restraints to prevent the client from removing the tube

    b. Do not place plastic tubes in ice because they will become stiff and inflexible, causing trauma to mucous membranes; rubber tubes can be placed in ice for 10 to 15 minutes to ease their insertion

    c. Keep the head of the client's bed elevated 30 degrees after tube insertion

    d. Check tube placement at least every 4 hours, or according to institution policy

    e. Notify the physician of increased or continued client vomiting or abdominal distention, failure of tube to drain after irrigation or repositioning of the client, or any unusual drainage

    f. If the tube is not draining, advance or withdraw it slightly; then reassess its placement

    g. Check for the return of bowel function every 4 hours by listening for bowel sounds, assessing for abdominal distention, and asking if the client has passed flatus

    h. Frequently assess nostrils for discharge and irritation, and change the tape anchoring the tube at least once daily or whenever it becomes soiled

    i. Clean the tube and the client's nostrils with a cotton-tipped applicator moistened with warm water

    j. Apply a water-soluble lubricant to the nostrils and petrolatum to the lips to prevent drying

    k. Do not give the client anything by mouth unless ordered by the physician; provide frequent mouth care, since the mouth will become dry as the client breathes through it

    l. Check with the physician about allowing sips of water, small ice chips, gargling solutions, throat lozenges, hard candy, or chewing gum to increase saliva

    m. If the tube is used for feedings, check placement before each feeding; for continuous feedings, check at least every 4 hours, or according to institution policy; for intermittent feedings, check for residual stomach contents from the previous feeding and either replace contents into the stomach or consult the physician if residual is large; check the physician's order or institution policy for the amount of residual to be reinserted or withheld

C. NG tube irrigation

  1. General information

    a. Irrigation is the flushing of an NG tube with a small amount of prescribed solution, usually isotonic normal saline, to maintain tube patency

    b. An NG tube can become clogged with clotted blood, tissue debris, or thickened feeding formula

    c. Water is contraindicated as an irrigating solution because it can cause an electrolyte imbalance (for example, alkalosis may result from removal of acid gastric contents)

  2. Purpose

    a. To maintain tube patency

    b. To reestablish tube patency if drainage slows or stops

  3. Procedure: Irrigating an NG tube

    a. Review the institution's policy, check the client's condition and diagnosis, and obtain a physician's order, if required

    b. Explain the procedure to the client

    c. Assemble equipment: suction device, irrigating set (basin and bulb syringe), irrigating solution (normal saline or as specified in the physician's order), plug or clamp, and clean disposable gloves

    d. Open the irrigation set, and pour saline solution into the basin

e. Wash hands and don gloves
f. Place a protective pad or towel under the end of the tube; unclamp the tube or disconnect it from the suction device or continuous feeding formula
g. Check tube placement by using a syringe to aspirate gastric contents; if no contents are aspirated, inject 10 cc of air while listening with a stethoscope over the epigastric area
h. Fill the bulb syringe with 30 to 50 ml of saline solution
i. Insert the syringe into the tube, and slowly inject the prescribed amount of irrigating solution; if you have difficulty injecting the solution into the tube, suspect an obstruction; check the tubing for kinks or reposition the client or tube and try again
j. Gently aspirate the solution and repeat until the ordered amount of solution has been used
k. Reconnect the tube to the suction device, continuous feeding formula, or clamp; for a Salem sump tube, inject 10 cc of air into the vent lumen (the smaller lumen) after reconnecting the tube to suction
l. Observe the drainage system for several minutes to ensure its proper functioning
4. Documentation
a. Record how tube placement was confirmed, the time of irrigation, and the amount and type of solution used and drainage returned
b. Document patency of the system after irrigation
c. Note on the intake and output sheet the amount of fluid instilled and drained
d. Chart nursing assessments before and after irrigation
e. Record any evidence of tube malfunction, such as abdominal distention, decreased or absent drainage flow, abdominal discomfort or pain, or vomiting
5. Nursing considerations
a. Avoid frequent irrigation, which can lead to electrolyte imbalance or metabolic acidosis; use other nursing measures, such as repositioning the client or NG tube
b. To facilitate drainage from the tube, encourage the client to turn from side to side and, when permitted, to ambulate
c. Regularly check the drainage system to verify its proper functioning
d. Empty the drainage container every 8 hours or whenever it becomes three-quarters full
e. Always verify tube placement before irrigation

D. NG tube removal
1. General information
a. An NG tube is usually temporary
b. A nurse removes the tube on a physician's orders; in some circumstances, institution policy may prohibit a nurse from removing it

    c. The physician may order that the tube be clamped for a time so that the client can be assessed for problems, such as vomiting

    d. When the tube is clamped, the physician may order a trial fluid intake with water, tea, or broth

2. Purpose

    a. To discontinue gastric decompression in a client whose normal gastrointestinal function has returned

    b. To insert into another nostril if the first becomes irritated

    c. To discontinue enteral feedings in a client who can resume normal eating

3. Procedure: Removing an NG tube

    a. Check the physician's order for time of removal and any specific instructions for clamping or unclamping the tube

    b. Explain the procedure to the client

    c. Assemble supplies: tissues, clean disposable gloves, plastic bag, waterproof pad

    d. Wash hands and don gloves

    e. Place a protective pad or towel under the end of the tube

    f. Turn off suctioning or continuous feeding device, and disconnect the NG tube from suction tubing

    g. Remove tape from the client's nose, and unpin the tube from the client's gown

    h. Clamp, plug, or pinch tubing with the fingers; then ask the client to take a long, slow, deep breath, and quickly and continuously remove the tube

    i. Place the tube in a plastic bag and discard it

    j. Provide tissues for the client to blow his nose, and help him wash his face

    k. Remove any additional equipment, such as suction apparatus, from the bedside; measure the amount of drainage in the container, and clean the apparatus according to institution policy; empty and rinse the drainage bottle

4. Documentation

    a. Record the client's tolerance of periodic tube clamping ordered by the physician

    b. Note the time of tube removal

    c. Document nursing assessments, such as abdominal status, presence or absence of bowel sounds, passing of flatus, and the client's response to the tube removal

5. Nursing considerations

    a. Continue regular assessment of the client's gastrointestinal status

    b. Closely monitor bowel sounds for changes

    c. Evaluate the client's ability to tolerate oral feedings

    d. Keep an accurate fluid intake and output sheet

E. Enteral tube feeding
1. General information
   a. For enteral tube feedings, the nurse instills liquid food preparations into the client's stomach or small intestine through a tube
   b. The procedure is also called tube feeding or gavage
2. Types
   a. *Intermittent bolus feedings* deliver 250 to 300 ml of formula over 15 to 30 minutes, usually through a large-lumen tube, such as a Levin tube
   b. *Intermittent gravity drip feedings* deliver 250 to 400 ml of formula at a prescribed flow rate over a prescribed time, four to six times a day
   c. *Continuous drip feedings* deliver formula at a constant rate over 24 hours through a tube with a smaller lumen, such as a Keofeed tube; usually, the tube is connected to a pump that controls the flow rate
3. Purpose: to provide nutrition for a client who cannot or will not eat or swallow a sufficient amount of food and fluids
4. Procedure: Administering an intermittent bolus feeding
   a. Check the physician's order and the nursing care plan for the timing, amount, method, and correct feeding formula
   b. Assemble supplies: 20- to 50-ml syringe or bulb syringe, emesis basin, measuring container, formula, warm water, feeding pump (optional), calibrated plastic bag, and tubing
   c. Check the formula's expiration date
   d. Bring the formula to room temperature, and measure the amount needed; if feedings are to be left hanging for 3 to 4 hours (or according to manufacturer's recommendations), cool the formula with ice chips
   e. Help the client into a high Fowler's position or an elevated right sidelying position to facilitate emptying of the stomach
   f. Wash hands and don gloves
   g. Check tube placement; aspirate all stomach contents and measure the aspirated amount; if 50 ml or more of undigested formula is withdrawn from an adult (10 ml or more from a child), check with the charge nurse; at some institutions, a feeding is withheld when a specified amount of formula remains in the stomach; in other institutions, the amount of formula withdrawn is subtracted from the total feeding; gastric contents can be reinstilled into the stomach
   h. Clamp or pinch off the NG tube, remove the bulb from the bulb syringe, and connect the syringe to the tube; pour the formula into the syringe
   i. Unclamp the NG tube and allow the formula to flow slowly; adjust the rate by raising or lowering the syringe; pinch or clamp the NG tube to stop the flow if the client is uncomfortable or complains of cramps
   j. When the feeding is almost complete (5 to 10 ml left in syringe), add 60 ml of water to the syringe to rinse the tube before the formula has completely drained from the syringe
   k. Clamp or pinch the NG tube before removing the syringe
   l. After the feeding, ask the client to remain in a high Fowler's position for 30 minutes to facilitate stomach emptying

m. If equipment will be reused, wash thoroughly with soap and water and dry; change equipment every 24 hours or according to institution policy
5. Procedure: Administering an intermittent gravity drip feeding
   a. Prepare the client and formula as for a bolus feeding
   b. Prepare the feeding system, and clamp the feeding tube
   c. Hang a burette (institution-prepared open container) or commercial prefilled bottle or bag on an infusion pole about 12″ (30 cm) above the NG tube insertion site
   d. Squeeze the container's drip chamber to fill it one-third to one-half of its capacity
   e. Open the clamp, run formula through the tubing, and reclamp
   f. Confirm tube placement
   g. Attach the feeding system to the NG tube and regulate the drip rate to deliver formula over the prescribed time
   h. When the feeding is almost complete, use the bulb syringe to flush the NG tube with 60 ml of water
6. Procedure: Administering a continuous drip feeding
   a. Prepare the client and formula as for intermittent gravity drip feeding
   b. Follow the intermittent gravity drip procedure to prepare the feeding system
   c. To check NG tube placement, interrupt the feeding; then aspirate and measure stomach contents; follow institution policy for the amount of aspirated feeding
   d. Flush the NG tube with 30 to 50 ml of water to maintain tube patency
   e. Connect a new feeding system and regulate the flow rate
7. Documentation
   a. Document the time feeding started and the amount, type, and duration of the feeding
   b. Note the client's response to the feeding
   c. Record the amount of formula and water on the intake and output sheet
8. Nursing considerations
   a. Administer intermittent bolus feedings slowly and assess the client carefully because these feedings can cause cramping, vomiting, aspiration, flatus, and diarrhea
   b. Know that intermittent gravity drip feedings can be given through an NG tube, a gastrostomy, or a jejunostomy for clients with normal gastrointestinal function
   c. Check NG tube placement carefully to avoid aspiration of formula into the airway
   d. Be aware that continuous drip feedings are recommended for seriously ill or comatose clients because of the risk of aspiration from bolus feedings
   e. Check NG tube placement every 4 hours, when a new bag or bottle of formula is ordered, or according to institution policy

F. Enema administration
1. General information
   a. During illness or hospitalization, a client is at risk for changes in bowel function
   b. Constipation commonly results from a change in routine, the stress of illness and hospitalization, or immobility
   c. An enema is a solution injected into the rectum to stimulate peristalsis and remove flatus or feces by distending or irritating the bowel
   d. Before giving an enema, a nurse helps the client use natural methods to promote evacuation of feces and flatus, such as sitting with the thighs flexed, taking adequate time (the nurse ensures privacy), eating high-fiber foods, increasing fluid intake, and exercising
   e. Some enemas are commercially prepared (oil retention or hypertonic enemas); others are made of soapsuds (cleansing enemas), saline solution, or tap water
   f. The amount of solution used depends on the physician's order, the type of enema, and the client's age and size
   g. The size of the rectal catheter used depends on the client (a #22 to #30 French rectal tube for an adult, a #12 to #18 French for a child)
2. Purpose
   a. To relieve constipation
   b. To soften and remove fecal impactions
   c. To empty the bowel in preparation for X-ray, surgery, certain diagnostic procedures, or childbirth
3. Procedure: Administering an enema
   a. Read the physician's order for the type of enema to administer, the amount of solution to use, and the frequency of administration
   b. Gather equipment: enema container, tubing and clamp, bath thermometer, lubricant, waterproof pad, bath blanket, toilet tissue and bedpan, clean disposable gloves, washcloth, towel, basin, I.V. pole (optional), and prepackaged enema, if used
   c. Place the client in Sims' position (left sidelying), with the right leg flexed; place a child or a client with poor sphincter control on a padded bedpan in a dorsal recumbent position
   d. Put a waterproof pad under the client's hips and buttocks
   e. Drape the client with a bath blanket, exposing only the buttocks, and place the bedpan on the bed, close to the client
   f. Wash hands, don gloves, and pour the prescribed solution into the enema container
   g. Remove the protective cap from the rectal tube tip, open the tubing clamp, and allow a small amount of solution to flow into the bedpan; reclamp and lubricate the tip
   h. Separate the client's buttocks to expose the anus
   i. Instruct the client to take a deep breath; insert the rectal tube into the anus, directing it toward the umbilicus

      j. Unclamp the tubing and allow the solution to flow slowly into the rectum; if using a disposable enema, squeeze the enema container until the appropriate quantity of the solution has been instilled

      k. Hold the enema solution approximately 18″ (45 cm) above the bowel as the solution is flowing; stop the flow if the client complains of severe cramping or of excess fullness

      l. Clamp the tubing, remove the rectal tube, and wipe the anus with toilet tissue

      m. Remove gloves and help the client to the toilet, commode, or bedpan to expel the solution

      n. Don gloves and help the client wash and dry the perianal area

      o. Discard disposable enema equipment in a proper container or rinse with soap and water if it is reusable

      p. Before emptying the bedpan or flushing the toilet, examine the solution and feces to determine if stool has been evacuated or fluid has been retained

4. Documentation

      a. Document the type of enema administered and the amount of solution used

      b. Record characteristics of the expelled solution and the color, amount, consistency, and characteristics of the feces

      c. Document unusual or unexpected outcomes, such as retention of enema solution or pain

      d. Note the client's tolerance of the procedure

5. Nursing considerations

      a. Use care when inserting a rectal tube in a client with hemorrhoids; use generous amounts of lubricant to reduce friction when passing the tube

      b. Never give an enema to a client suspected of having appendicitis or bowel obstruction

      c. If the client cannot control his external sphincter, place him on a bedpan during the entire procedure

      d. Do not administer an enema when the client is sitting on the toilet because curved rectal tubing can abrade the rectal wall

      e. If the physician's order states "enema until clear," repeat large-volume enemas until the client passes clear fluid containing no feces; a client is usually given no more than three enemas because fluid and electrolyte balance can be disturbed; check institution policy

G. Rectal tube insertion

1. General information

      a. Excessive flatus in the gastrointestinal tract leads to distention (stretching and inflating of the intestines)

      b. Distention can result from anesthesia, narcotics, dietary changes, or reduced activity; distention after surgery is uncomfortable for the client

      c. A tube placed in the rectum allows flatus to be removed by siphon

   d. Rubber or flexible plastic rectal tubes are available in sizes #22 to #30 French for adults and #12 to #18 French for children
2. Purpose
   a. To remove flatus from the lower gastrointestinal tract
   b. To relieve abdominal distention
   c. To increase client comfort
3. Procedure: Inserting a rectal tube
   a. Read the physician's order and the nursing care plan
   b. Assemble equipment: rectal tube, small plastic bag or specimen container, waterproof pad, clean disposable gloves, and tape
   c. Place the rectal tube's distal end in a plastic bag and secure it with tape or a rubber band, or place it through the opening in the specimen container lid and secure it with tape; cut a small slit to vent the bag or container
   d. Wash hands and don gloves
   e. Help the client to a left sidelying position; drape him with a bath blanket, with buttocks exposed; and place a waterproof pad under the buttocks
   f. Lubricate the tip of the rectal tube and insert it 4″ to 6″ (10 to 15 cm) into the rectum, toward the umbilicus
   g. Secure the tube with two strips of tape, and leave it in place for 15 to 20 minutes
   h. Remove the tube and wash and dry the client's anal area if needed
   i. Remove gloves and wash hands
   j. Clean reusable tubing; discard disposable tubing
4. Documentation
   a. Record the time of tube insertion and removal
   b. Note the amount, color, and consistency of any feces passed
   c. Document the presence or absence of distention
5. Nursing considerations
   a. Reinsert the rectal tube, if needed, every 2 to 3 hours
   b. Assess abdominal distention and client discomfort before and after tube insertion
   c. Help the client to change position frequently and to ambulate, if permitted, while the tube is in place

H. Fecal impaction removal
   1. General information
      a. Fecal impaction occurs when feces are too hard or too large to be passed
      b. The client expresses discomfort and a desire to defecate but cannot; small amounts of liquid stool are passed, and abdominal distention may occur
      c. Breaking up and removing the fecal mass is uncomfortable and embarrassing for the client

      d. Attempts to remove the fecal mass can cause irritation and bleeding or stimulate the vagus nerve, which can lead to a reflex slowing of the heart

  2. Purpose
      a. To remove a large or hard fecal mass from the rectum
      b. To promote the return of normal bowel function
      c. To increase client comfort

  3. Procedure: Removing a fecal impaction
      a. Read the physician's order, keeping in mind that a client with a cardiac condition or spinal cord injury may be at risk for vagal stimulation; consult institution policy
      b. Assemble equipment: clean disposable gloves, lubricant, waterproof pad, bedpan, toilet tissue, washcloth, towel, and soap
      c. Prepare the client as for an enema or rectal tube insertion
      d. Don gloves; lubricate the index finger, and insert it into the rectum toward the umbilicus
      e. Gently loosen the fecal mass from the rectal wall; break feces into small pieces and remove them
      f. Allow the client to rest
      g. Assess the client's heart rate; stop the procedure if the rate drops or the rhythm changes
      h. Help the client to the bedpan or toilet
      i. Remove gloves, clean equipment, and wash hands
      j. Administer an enema, if ordered

  4. Documentation
      a. Record the client's response to the procedure, and report any adverse effects
      b. Document the amount, color, and consistency of the stool removed and any stool passed after manual removal

  5. Nursing considerations
      a. Administer an enema after disimpaction, if ordered
      b. Inform the client of dietary measures to promote bowel evacuation

I. Enterostomy pouch application
  1. General information
      a. An enterostomy is any surgical procedure that results in an artificial opening (stoma) in a portion of the intestine through the abdominal wall
      b. Two types of enterostomy are ileostomy and colostomy
      c. The location of the enterostomy determines the consistency of the client's stool; an ileostomy and ascending colon colostomy produce frequent liquid stools that contain digestive enzymes; a colostomy of the transverse colon produces thicker and formed stools; a sigmoid colostomy produces stools formed like those from the rectum

  2. Purpose
      a. To protect the skin around the stoma from erythema, excoriation, infection, and fistula (abnormal opening)

      b. To contain drainage and odors so the client feels socially acceptable

      c. To protect the client's clothing

      d. To collect drainage or stool for assessment

3. Procedure: Applying an enterostomy pouch

      a. Check the physician's order and the nursing care plan for client-specific instructions

      b. Explain the procedure to the client and family members; encourage the client to participate in any way possible

      c. Assemble and prepare equipment and supplies: clean pouch (drainable pouch except for a descending or sigmoid colostomy), pouch clamp, skin barriers (such as Skin Gel or Skin Prep), basin with warm water, skin cleanser or mild soap, plastic disposable trash bags, clean disposable gloves, bath blanket, washcloth, and towel

      d. Discuss with the client the best time to change the pouch (immediately if it is leaking); consider mealtimes, medication administration, and client comfort

      e. Place the client in high Fowler's or standing position, drape a bath blanket over the client, and fanfold bedding to the foot of the bed

      f. Prepare a clean pouch: trace a circle ⅙″ to ⅛″ (2 to 3 mm) larger than the stoma on the paper covering the adhesive backing of the faceplate, cut the stoma pattern, and apply cement or a double-faced adhesive disk, according to the type of pouch used

      g. Prepare the occlusive skin barrier, ensuring that the barrier opening is the same size as the stoma to prevent the stoma from touching the skin; if using a karaya ring, moisten the ring until it becomes sticky; if using Stomahesive or Reliaseal, cut an opening to the stoma as for the pouch

      h. Empty and gently remove the old pouch

      i. Wash the client's skin with a cleanser or soap and water; remove all secretions, rinse, and blot dry

      j. Observe the condition and color of the skin and stoma; note any edema or ulceration

      k. Apply an occlusive skin barrier; if not using an occlusive barrier, spray the skin with a skin barrier (such as Skin Prep), allow it to dry, and spray again

      l. Center and apply a clean pouch directly on the skin or karaya ring, away from fresh incision lines

      m. Press adhesive around the stoma to form a seal; avoid wrinkles, which can cause leakage

      n. Fold the bottom edges of the pouch and secure the end with a clamp

      o. Apply hypoallergenic tape, if needed, to faceplate edges over the skin barrier; attach a belt to the faceplate of the pouch (optional)

      p. Dispose of the old appliance, clean reusable items, remove gloves, and wash hands

4. Documentation

      a. Record the type of pouch and skin barrier used and when the pouch was applied or changed

       b. Log the amount, color, and consistency of stool

       c. Note the condition of the skin and stoma

       d. Record the client's participation in self-care

   5. Nursing considerations

       a. Check with the enterostomal therapist about equipment and modifications in the care plan; barriers and pouches used in ostomy care are selected on the basis of chemical composition and consistency of drainage, surgical construction of the stoma, and firmness and contour of the abdomen

       b. Empty pouches when one-third to one-half full of feces or flatus to prevent destruction of the pouch seal

       c. Notify the physician immediately if necrosis or vascular problems develop (for example, if the stoma appears dark, dusky-colored, or black)

       d. Be aware that a colostomy may not drain for the first 5 days

       e. If the client is ambulatory, apply the pouch downward; otherwise, apply at an angle over the iliac crest

       f. Know that pouches applied with adhesive can be left in place for several days, unless leakage or skin irritation occurs

       g. Change the pouch every 4 to 7 days if the client is not irrigating the colostomy

J. Colostomy irrigation

   1. General information

       a. In colostomy irrigation, fluid is instilled to remove fecal contents

       b. The procedure should be performed at the same time every day or every other day, as ordered, and is simple enough for a client to perform

       c. Colostomy irrigation is routinely performed for a client with a descending or sigmoid colostomy to empty the bowel once daily and to eliminate the need for a pouch

       d. The procedure is rarely needed for a client with an ileostomy because drainage is liquid and frequent, except when blockage occurs; gentle lavage is used because of the danger of perforation

   2. Purpose

       a. To establish a regular pattern of bowel elimination

       b. To expel stool from the colon

   3. Procedure: Irrigating a colostomy

       a. Review the physician's order and nursing care plan

       b. Assemble equipment: washcloth and warm water, water container with cone or #18 French catheter, 500 to 1,000 ml of water at 105° to 110° F (40.5° to 43.4° C), belt and irrigating sleeve, clean pouch, skin barriers, lubricant, plastic bag, I.V. pole, and clean disposable gloves

       c. Discuss the procedure with the client

       d. Wash hands, don gloves, and remove and discard the pouch

       e. Clean the client's skin as for changing a pouch, and place an irrigation sleeve over the stoma

      f. Lubricate the catheter or cone, and fill the irrigation container with 500 to 1,000 ml of tepid water; hang the container on the I.V. pole and run fluid through the tubing

      g. Help the client sit on the toilet or a chair in front of the toilet

      h. Insert the cone or catheter gently but firmly into the stoma about 2″ to 4″ (5 to 10 cm); never force the insertion

      i. Start water flow slowly, and allow it to run into the stoma for 10 to 15 minutes; keep the irrigation container level with the client's shoulder

      j. Pause when the client has cramps or if reflux occurs; clamp the tube and have the client take slow, deep breaths to relax

      k. Close off or fold over the top of the irrigation sleeve while the client remains seated, allowing most of the solution to return

      l. Rinse the sleeve with water, dry the bottom, and close the end; let the client walk or resume other activities for 30 to 45 minutes while the remainder of the solution is expelled

      m. Remove the sleeve, clean the client's skin and stoma, and apply a new pouch and skin barrier

      n. Rinse and dry the irrigation sleeve

      o. Remove gloves and wash hands

4. Documentation

      a. Record the time of irrigation, the amount and type of solution used, and results obtained

      b. Note the condition of the skin and stoma

      c. Document the client's reaction to and degree of participation in the procedure

5. Nursing considerations

      a. Reassure the client that a small amount of bleeding around the stoma is normal

      b. Discontinue irrigation until stool thickens in a client with diarrhea

      c. Be aware that an irrigation cone is safer to use than a catheter because it is less likely to perforate the colon

      d. If water does not flow easily into the stoma, change the cone's angle or position, check for kinks in the tubing, and ask the client to relax and take deep breaths

Points to Remember

Water is not used to irrigate an NG tube because it may cause electrolyte imbalances.

Before administering an enema, the nurse should promote natural passage of feces by having the client sit with thighs flexed, providing privacy, and encouraging the client to drink fluids.

If the physician orders "enemas until clear" before surgery or diagnostic tests, administer a large-volume tap water, saline, or soapsuds enema one to three times until the returned fluid is free of feces.

Digital removal of a fecal impaction can stimulate the vagus nerve, resulting in slowing of the heart rate.

Signs of necrosis or vascular problems in a client with a colostomy should be reported to the physician.

Close fit of the barrier around the stoma prevents drainage from touching the skin and reduces the risk of skin irritation.

Glossary

Bolus — an amount of liquid food, fluid, or medication given at one time

Colostomy — surgical opening (stoma) between the colon and the body surface through which feces pass

Fecal impaction — retention of hard, dried stool in the colon or rectum

Gastric decompression — removal of fluid and gas through a tube by use of negative pressure or suction

Hemorrhoid — internal or external dilated blood vessel in the colon, rectum, or anal area

Peristalsis — contraction and relaxation of successive portions of the alimentary canal that moves food, fluid, and flatus forward

Glossary *(continued)*

Retention enema — solution (usually oil based) that is introduced into the lower bowel to soften feces and aid in feces expulsion

Salem sump tube — double-lumen tube usually made of plastic; the larger lumen drains stomach contents while the smaller lumen, or air vent, permits inflow of air, preventing suction if the tube sticks to the stomach wall

Tube feeding — administration of nutrients through a tube into the stomach

Administering Medication

Learning Objectives

After studying this section, the reader should be able to:

• List the five "rights" of safe medication administration.

• Cite the safety checks common to administration of all drugs.

• Review factors that the nurse should assess before drug administration.

• Identify common intradermal, subcutaneous, and intramuscular injection sites.

• Discuss the procedure for administering medication by each route.

• Describe the nursing responsibilities of medication administration.

VIII. Administering Medication

A. Introduction

1. Medication administration, a dependent nursing function, involves preparing and giving drugs ordered by a physician to a client for therapeutic purposes
2. Safe and accurate medication administration is one of the nurse's major responsibilities
3. A primary means of therapy, medication can be harmful if administered improperly
4. Before giving any medication, the nurse must:
   a. Know the drug's prescribed dose, method of administration, actions, expected therapeutic effect, possible interactions with other drugs, and adverse effects
   b. Know and use the institution's administration procedures for the client's welfare and the nurse's legal protection
   c. Review the physician's order for completeness: the client's name, date of the order, name of the drug, dose, route, time of administration, and the physician's signature
   d. Discuss the medication and its actions with the client; recheck the medication order if the client disagrees with the dose or the physician's order
   e. Check the physician's order against the client's medication administration record for accuracy
5. To ensure the client's safety, the nurse adheres to the five "rights" of medication administration:
   a. Right drug
   b. Right dose
   c. Right client
   d. Right route
   e. Right time
6. The patient also has the right to know about the medication he is receiving and the right to refuse it.
7. Commonly used administration routes are *oral* (usually absorbed in the gastrointestinal tract), *topical* (applied to the skin or mucous membranes), and *parenteral* (administered by injection with a needle)
8. Medication can also be instilled into the eye or ear or administered by suppository
9. Medication may be given on a regular schedule, as a one-time dose, or as needed (p.r.n.)

B. Oral medication administration

1. General information
   a. Is the easiest and most desirable type of drug to administer
   b. Is commonly called P.O. medication (from the Latin *per os,* meaning "through the mouth")

    c. Has the slowest onset of action because it is absorbed through the gastric mucosa into the bloodstream for a systemic effect

    d. Can have a local effect (for example, antacids)

    e. Is supplied in the form of tablets, capsules, enteric-coated tablets, liquids, syrups, and suspensions

    f. Is contraindicated in a client who is vomiting or cannot swallow food or fluids, who is having gastric suctioning, or who lacks mental awareness

2. Purpose

    a. To provide safe, effective drug therapy with minimal complications and discomfort

    b. To provide a convenient route for drug therapy

3. Procedure: Administering oral medication

    a. Wash hands

    b. Take the medication cart to the client's room, if possible, to reduce the chances of making an error, and remove the medication container from the cart

    c. Compare the label on the bottle or package wrapper with the medication administration record *(first safety check)*

    d. Correctly calculate the dose; check with another nurse if unsure of the calculation or when administering certain drugs, such as narcotic analgesics

    e. Open the bottle or package, and pour solid oral medication into the lid of the container and then into the medicine cup; place into a separate cup any medication (such as digoxin) that requires client assessment before administration; place individually wrapped medications in the cup

    f. Remove the bottle lid from a liquid oral medication and place the lid upside down to prevent contamination; pour medication from the bottle—with the label facing up and covered by the palm—into a medicine cup placed on a firm surface or held in the hand at eye level; read the fluid level at the lowest point of the meniscus; wipe the bottle's lip before replacing the lid

    g. Compare the drug label on the bottle or package wrapper with the client's medication administration record before placing medication in the cup *(second safety check)*

    h. Read the label again before replacing the medication bottle; for wrapped single-dose drugs, read the label again in the client's room after identifying the client *(third safety check)*

    i. Carry medication to the client's room on a cart or tray

    j. Compare identification on the client's bracelet—including name, room, and bed number—with the medication record

    k. Help the client to a sitting position if permitted

    l. Perform assessments as required, such as checking the client's apical pulse rate before administering digoxin

    m. Give the medicine cup to the client; some clients prefer to swallow more than one pill at a time, while others swallow a single pill at a time

   n. Provide a glass of water, and make sure the client swallows the
       medication; then discard the medicine cup
   o. Observe the client for drug action and adverse reactions; know the best
       time to evaluate the drug's effects
4. Procedure: Administering a controlled substance orally
   a. Unlock the narcotics cupboard, drawer, or box, and retrieve the
       appropriate narcotic container
   b. Count the number of pills, ampules, or cartridges in the container; check
       the accuracy of the count against the narcotics sign-out sheet; inform the
       charge nurse before proceeding if the count is incorrect
   c. Remove the drug from the container
   d. Sign for the drug on the narcotics sign-out sheet (some institutions
       require a second signature if a portion of the drug is discarded or if a
       student is administering the drug)
   e. Lock the narcotic cupboard, drawer, or box
   f. Continue the procedure as for oral medication administration
5. Procedure: Administering sublingual or buccal medication
   a. Follow the procedure for oral medication administration
   b. Place the drug under the client's tongue for sublingual administration, or
       instruct the client to do so; place buccal medication between the client's
       cheek and gum
   c. Tell the client that he must not swallow the medication or drink liquids
       until the drug is absorbed
6. Documentation
   a. Complete institution medication administration forms as soon as possible
       after administration
   b. Record the drug name, dose, route, and time administered
   c. Sign full name and title abbreviation
   d. Document in the nurses' notes or the client's record the client's response
       to the drug and any unusual reaction (or, if applicable, note whether and
       why the drug was withheld or the client refused to take it)
7. Nursing considerations
   a. If a client has difficulty swallowing tablets, check with the pharmacy to
       determine if the medication can be crushed or substituted with a liquid
   b. Do not offer water after administering cough syrup or antacids to prevent
       interference with the medication's intended action
   c. Mix crushed pills or liquids with a small amount of food or liquid,
       unless contraindicated by the client's diet order
   d. Use a syringe to measure small doses of liquid medications accurately
   e. Shake suspensions before pouring to mix the drug thoroughly
   f. Have one nurse ending a shift and one nurse starting the next shift count
       all narcotics; check the accuracy of narcotics sign-out sheets at the end
       of each shift
   g. When a narcotic container is empty, send the container and sign-out
       sheet to the pharmacy for replacement

SYRINGE AND NEEDLE SPECIFICATIONS

TYPE OF INJECTION	SYRINGE SIZE	NEEDLE GAUGE AND LENGTH
Intradermal	1 ml tuberculin	25G to 27G; ⅜" to ½" (0.9 to 1 cm)
Subcutaneous	1 to 3 ml	25G to 27G; ⅜" to ⅝" (0.9 to 1.6 cm)
Intramuscular	1 to 5 ml	23G to 25G for use in a small muscle or for an infant, 18G to 23G for an adult; ⅝" to 1" (1.6 to 2.5 cm) for use in a small muscle or for an infant, 1" to 1½" (2.5 to 3.8 cm) for an adult

    h. When receiving a new supply of narcotic drugs, check the accuracy of the count, sign a receipt on receiving the drugs, and lock them in the narcotics cupboard, drawer, or box

    i. If a p.r.n. drug is ordered, assess the client to determine if he needs the drug (for example, if the physician's order states, "Give every 4 hours p.r.n. when temperature is above 101° F," determine when the client last had the drug, take his temperature, and (if the temperature is over 101°F), administer the drug only if 4 hours have elapsed since the last dose)

    j. Never administer medication poured by someone else

    k. Discard any unused medication, and notify the pharmacy; do not return it to the stock container

    l. Know that when a nurse discards any narcotic, another nurse must co-sign the narcotics sign-out sheet

C. Parenteral medication administration
  1. General information

    a. Is injected into body tissues with a needle and syringe

    b. Requires sterile technique to prevent local or systemic infection from introduction of pathogens into tissues

    c. Is preferred when administering a drug that the GI tract destroys or does not absorb

    d. Must be prepared or premixed in a syringe before administration; syringe size is determined by the amount of solution to be injected; needle size is determined by the injection site and the amount and type of medication to be given; needle length is determined by the depth of the injection (see *Syringe and needle specifications*)

    e. Is supplied in ampules, vials, dry powder (which must be mixed with sterile water or saline solution to make an injectable solution), and prefilled medication cartridges (see *Preparing parenteral medication,* pages 96 and 97)

PREPARING PARENTERAL MEDICATION

HOW SUPPLIED	PREPARATION INSTRUCTIONS
Ampule	• Flick the upper stem of the ampule to bring medication down into the main portion of the ampule. • Place gauze around the ampule neck. • Hold the body of the ampule upright in one hand, with the top between the thumb and finger of the other hand. • Break off the top, moving it away from yourself, using a snapping motion with firm, steady pressure. • Insert an uncapped, sterile needle that is attached to the syringe into the ampule, being careful not to touch the rim of the ampule. • Aspirate medication from the ampule by pulling back on the syringe plunger. • If a filter needle is used to remove medication from the ampule, replace it with an appropriate needle for the injection.
Vial	• Rotate the vial between both hands to mix the drug. • Remove the protective metal cap. • Clean the rubber cap with an alcohol pad, using a circular motion. • Pull back on the plunger, and fill a syringe that is attached to a needle with an amount of air equal to the amount of drug to be withdrawn from the vial. • Insert the needle at an angle into the center of the vial stopper. • Inject the air into the vial above the fluid level. • Invert the vial and withdraw the correct dose of medication into the syringe. • Withdraw the needle from the vial. • Check for excess air by pointing the needle up, tapping the side of the syringe, and pushing on the plunger. • Change the needle if necessary.
Powdered drug in a vial	• Read the manufacturer's instructions and follow the directions for dilution and reconstitution. • Use sterile water or saline solution as a diluent. • Withdraw the recommended amount of diluent using the procedure for preparing medication from a vial. • Wipe the stopper from a powdered medication vial with an alcohol pad. • Add diluent to the powdered drug. • Rotate the vial to mix the powder and diluent. • Label a multidose vial with the date and time of reconstitution and the amount of drug in each milliliter of solution; then initial the label. • Prepare a syringe with reconstituted medication using the procedure for preparing medication from a vial.

PREPARING PARENTERAL MEDICATION *(continued)*	
HOW SUPPLIED	**PREPARATION INSTRUCTIONS**
Mixing medications in one syringe	• Maintain the sterility of each drug. • When two vials are used, wipe the top of each vial with an alcohol pad. • Inject air into each vial equal to the amount of drug to be withdrawn. • Insert the needle into one vial and withdraw the specified amount of medication. • Remove the needle from the first vial, insert it into the second vial, and invert the vial. • Withdraw the specified amount of medication, and remove the needle. • When withdrawing insulin from two vials, withdraw shorter-acting insulin into the syringe first. • When using one vial and one ampule, inject air into the vial equal to the amount of drug to be withdrawn; withdraw the drug from the vial first; then draw up medication from the ampule.

  f. Is injected *subcutaneously* (into the fatty tissue just below the dermis), *intramuscularly* (into the body of a muscle), *intradermally* (between the dermis and epidermis), or *intravenously* (into a vein)

  g. Is absorbed most rapidly when injected intravenously; least rapidly when injected subcutaneously or intradermally

2. Purpose

  a. To provide medication for quick absorption when oral route is inappropriate

  b. To promote client comfort

3. Procedure: Administering a subcutaneous injection

  a. Follow the procedure for oral medication administration: review the physician's order and the client's medication record, perform safety checks, and ensure proper client identification

  b. Assemble equipment: alcohol pads, vials or ampules of medication, sterile water or normal saline solution as diluent, syringe with appropriate needle, sterile gauze pads, and clean disposable gloves (required by some institutions because the client may bleed from the injection site)

  c. Prepare medication in the syringe

  d. Place the client in a position appropriate to the injection site selected (see *Subcutaneous injection sites,* page 98)

  e. Clean the injection site with an alcohol pad, using a circular motion

  f. Grasp the skin at the injection site firmly, using the thumb and forefinger of the nondominant hand to elevate the subcutaneous tissue, forming a fat fold

SUBCUTANEOUS INJECTION SITES

Subcutaneous injection sites (shown by the dotted areas) include the fat pads on the abdomen, upper hips, upper back, and lateral upper arms and thighs. For subcutaneous injections administered regularly, rotate injection sites. Choose one site in one area, move to the corresponding injection site in the next area, and so on. When returning to an area, choose a new site.

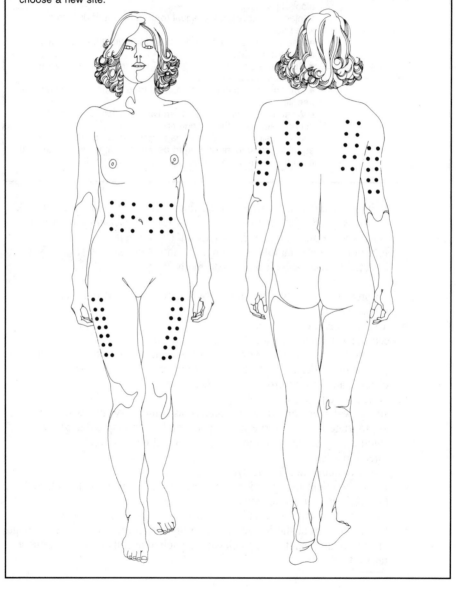

g. Holding the syringe like a dart between the thumb and forefinger of the dominant hand, insert the needle quickly at a 45- or 90-degree angle (the angle depends on the site and the amount of subcutaneous tissue)

h. Release the skin, hold the syringe barrel, and aspirate by pulling back on the plunger; if blood enters the syringe, withdraw and discard the needle, and prepare a new syringe and medication; if no blood is drawn, inject the medication slowly

i. Withdraw the needle and massage the site with an alcohol pad

j. Discard the uncapped needle and syringe in a safety container

k. Evaluate the client's response to the medication after 15 to 30 minutes

4. Procedure: Administering an intramuscular injection

a. Follow the procedure for oral medication administration: review the physician's order and the client's medication record, perform safety checks, and ensure proper client identification

b. Assemble equipment as for a subcutaneous injection

c. Prepare medication in the syringe

d. Select the injection site according to anatomic landmarks (see *Locating intramuscular injection sites,* pages 100 and 101)

e. Clean the site with an alcohol pad, using a circular motion from inside to outside

f. Spread skin at the injection site taut between the thumb and forefinger; for a child or an elderly client, grasp the muscle between fingers and thumb to increase muscle mass and help place the needle in the muscle

g. Insert the needle at a 90-degree angle, using a quick, darting motion

h. Aspirate by pulling back on the plunger; if blood enters the syringe, discard the needle and prepare a new syringe and medication; if no blood is drawn, inject the medication slowly

i. If using the Z-track method, pull the skin laterally away from the injection site; insert the needle at a 90-degree angle, wait 10 seconds after injecting the medication, and simultaneously withdraw the needle and release the skin

j. Massage the site with an alcohol pad; with the Z-track method, apply light pressure or pat with a pad

5. Procedure: Administering an intradermal injection

a. Explain to the client that the injection causes a bleb (akin to a mosquito bite or small blister) that will disappear quickly; advise that redness, swelling (induration), or hardness may appear later and will be assessed in 24 to 48 hours

b. Prepare the medication in the syringe

c. Select an appropriate injection site (free from discoloration, rash, or trauma); for example, intradermal skin testing for tuberculosis (PPD) is usually done on the inner forearm

d. Clean the site with an alcohol pad, using a circular motion

e. Hold the client's forearm in the palm, and grasp the client's inner forearm with thumb and fingers; gently pull the skin of the inner forearm taut

LOCATING INTRAMUSCULAR INJECTION SITES

Deltoid. To locate the densest area of muscle and avoid major nerves and blood vessels, first find the lower edge of the acromial process and the point on the lateral arm in line with the axilla. Insert the needle 1″ to 2″ (3 to 5 cm) below the acromial process, usually two to three fingerbreadths.

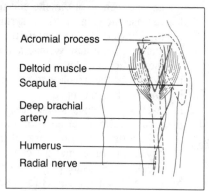

Acromial process

Deltoid muscle

Scapula

Deep brachial artery

Humerus

Radial nerve

Dorsogluteal (upper outer corner of the gluteus maximus). Restrict injections to the area above and outside the diagonal line drawn from the posterior superior iliac spine to the greater trochanter of the femur. Another method is to divide the buttock into quadrants, and inject in the upper outer quadrant, about 2″ to 3″ (5 to 8 cm) below the iliac crest.

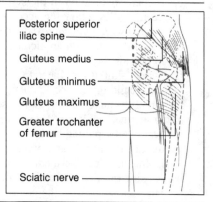

Posterior superior iliac spine

Gluteus medius

Gluteus minimus

Gluteus maximus

Greater trochanter of femur

Sciatic nerve

Ventrogluteal (gluteus medius and gluteus minimus). Locate the greater trochanter of the femur with the heel of the hand. Then spread the index and middle fingers to form a V from the anterior superior iliac spine to the farthest point along the iliac crest you can reach. Insert the needle into the area between the fingers.

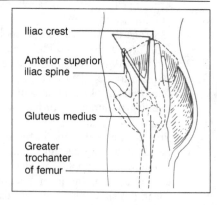

Iliac crest

Anterior superior iliac spine

Gluteus medius

Greater trochanter of femur

LOCATING INTRAMUSCULAR INJECTION SITES *(continued)*

Vastus lateralis. Use the lateral muscle of the quadriceps group, along that length of muscle from a handbreadth below the greater trochanter to a handbreadth above the knee. Insert the needle into the middle third of the muscle on a plane parallel to the surface on which the client is lying.

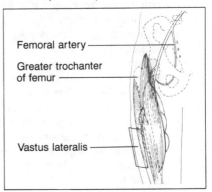

Femoral artery

Greater trochanter of femur

Vastus lateralis

---

     f. Insert the needle at a 10- to 15-degree angle, with the bevel of the needle up

     g. Do not aspirate

     h. Inject the test dose slowly until a bleb appears, indicating that the medication was injected within the dermis

     i. Withdraw the needle; do not massage the site

6. Documentation

     a. Record injection administration as soon as possible, using an institution form

     b. Chart the drug name, dose, route, site, time administered, nurse's initials, and signature by which the nurse identifies the initials on the client's medication record

     c. Document p.r.n., stat, and intradermal medications in the nurses' notes

     d. Record in the nurses' notes the client's response to the injection, including the client's report of pain relief or adverse reactions

7. Nursing considerations

     a. Interview the client to determine any history of allergies to injections

     b. Select an injection site free from scarring, tenderness, itching, inflammation, or hardness; use alternate sites to prevent tissue damage

     c. Read the medication label carefully to verify the correct drug, dose, and form

     d. If the client is an infant or child, do not use the dorsogluteal site (because of the potential for injury to the sciatic nerve) or the deltoid site (because of small muscle size)

     e. Use intramuscular injections to give medications, such as penicillin and paraldehyde, that irritate subcutaneous tissue

     f. Choose intramuscular injection sites carefully; injecting medication into areas where it cannot be absorbed can cause a sterile abscess

g. Reduce pain from an intramuscular injection by encouraging the client to relax the muscle, darting the needle into the skin and withdrawing it rapidly, and applying ice to produce a local anesthetic effect

h. When administering heparin subcutaneously, insert the needle at a 90-degree angle, and do not aspirate for blood or massage the injection site

i. Massage the area after injection unless contraindicated to help distribute the drug and promote its absorption

j. Know that the airlock (addition of 0.1 to 0.2 cc of air to the medication in the syringe before injection) is a controversial procedure; some experts believe that this small amount of air clears the needle of medication and ensures that all medication is injected; others believe the risk of error is increased when the amount of drug in the syringe hub and needle is given with the injection, because this is part of the syringe barrel calibration; the risk of error increases if all nurses do not use the same method

D. Topical medication administration
1. General information
   a. Is applied externally to the skin or mucous membranes
   b. Includes lotions, liniments, ointments, pastes, powders, creams, gels, jellies, aerosol sprays, and foams
   c. Requires use of sterile supplies and sterile technique when applied on open skin lesions
2. Purpose
   a. To facilitate absorption through the skin or mucous membranes
   b. To provide local anesthetic effect
   c. To stop, slow, or prevent microbial growth
3. Procedure: Applying topical medication
   a. Follow safety and identification steps for oral medication administration
   b. Assemble supplies: warm water, towel, sterile gauze squares or cotton, prescribed medication, tongue blade or clean disposable gloves, sterile gauze to hold medication taken from a stock jar (stock jars are not taken to the bedside) or to apply liquids, and sterile dressing and tape to place over the area, if indicated
   c. Wash hands and don gloves if necessary
   d. Determine whether the area to be treated is clean; wash with warm water or other solution as ordered; pat dry with towel or gauze
   e. Assess the area for redness, rash, swelling, or drainage
   f. Squeeze medication from the tube, take ointment from the jar with a tongue blade, or pour lotion onto the gauze
   g. Pat lotion onto the skin; spread a thin layer of ointment or cream, using a tongue blade or the fingers
   h. Apply a sterile dressing if indicated
   i. Clean and store all equipment properly; wash hands

4. Documentation
   a. Record the medication used, application site, time administered, and client response
   b. Chart skin appearance and any client complaints of discomfort or itching
   c. Assess and document relief of itching, burning, swelling, or other discomfort
5. Nursing considerations
   a. Know or research the properties of the topical medication
   b. Apply the correct topical preparation to the appropriate area
   c. Always use sterile technique when applying topical medication to open skin lesions
   d. Apply ointment or cream in a thin layer to prevent skin maceration

E. Eye medication administration
1. General information
   a. Is instilled as a sterile liquid, drops, or an ointment
   b. Is usually diluted (for example, less than 1% strength) and labeled for ophthalmic use
   c. Is supplied as a liquid in a plastic container also used for administration; as drops, in a container with a dropper; or as an ointment, in a small tube; in each case, the tip of the tube, the dropper, or the container is sterile
2. Purpose
   a. To provide a local effect
   b. To decrease intraocular pressure
   c. To dilate the pupils for an eye examination
3. Procedure: Instilling eye medication
   a. Follow safety and identification steps for oral medication administration; ensure that the medication is marked for ophthalmic use
   b. Assemble supplies: eye medication, facial tissue, and clean disposable gloves
   c. Wash hands and clean the client's eye as needed, wiping from the inner to outer canthus; wear gloves if the eye is infected
   d. Tilt the client's head back slightly, and ask the client to look up; provide tissues
   e. With a steady hand, hold a filled dropper ½" to ¾ " (1 to 2 cm) above the client's eye; hold eye ointment close to the lower lid
   f. Pull down on the client's cheek to expose the lower conjunctival sac
   g. Place the prescribed number of drops into the center of the conjunctival sac, or squeeze eye ointment from the tube into the lower conjunctival sac along the inside edge of the lower eyelid, starting at the inner canthus
   h. Do not allow the sterile tip of the dropper or tube to touch the eye
   i. Ask the client to close both eyes gently and blink; if ointment is used, ask the client to rotate the eyes to help distribute the medication over the eyeball

j. Use tissue or cotton balls to wipe excess medication from around the eyes; remove gloves and wash hands
4. Documentation
   a. Record the drug name, dose, route, site, time administered, and nurse's initials and signature
   b. Chart the condition of the eye and surrounding tissue in the nurses' notes
5. Nursing considerations
   a. Know the expected action of each medication
   b. Maintain sterility of the container and applicator tip to prevent infection
   c. Exert pressure on the bony prominences of the cheek or eyebrow and not on the eye to prevent eye trauma
   d. Avoid touching the conjunctival sac or cornea with an eye dropper or tube to prevent contamination

F. Ear medication administration
1. General information
   a. Is instilled as drops
   b. Is supplied in a plastic container also used to administer the drops or in a container with a dropper; ear medication is labeled for otic use
   c. Requires use of clean technique to instill medication; use of sterile technique is required if the tympanic membrane is damaged
2. Purpose
   a. To relieve ear pain
   b. To provide route for antibiotic medication
   c. To soften ear wax
3. Procedure: Instilling ear medication
   a. Follow safety and identification steps for oral medication administration; ensure that the medication is marked for otic use
   b. Gather supplies: prescribed ear drops, warm water (to bring the drops, if refrigerated, to room temperature), clean disposable gloves (if indicated), cotton ball
   c. Wash hands, and don gloves if the ear is draining
   d. Place the client in a sidelying position, with the affected ear up
   e. Fill the eardropper with the prescribed amount of medication
   f. Lift the pinna up and back (for an adult client), or draw the pinna gently downward and back (for a child)
   g. Hold the dropper slightly above the ear and administer medication; press a few times on the tragus to ease the flow of drops into the ear
   h. Insert a cotton ball at the ear opening; have the client remain in a sidelying position for 5 to 10 minutes to allow medication to flow into the ear canal and be distributed equally
   i. Assess the client for pain, discomfort, and ear discharge
   j. Wash hands
4. Documentation
   a. Record the drug name, dose, route, site, time administered, and nurse's initials and signature

      b. Document client complaints of pain or discomfort
      c. Chart characteristics of any ear drainage
  5. Nursing considerations
      a. Know the expected action of any drug administered
      b. Clean the pinna and external ear before administration if needed
      c. Before and after instilling drops, assess the pinna, external meatus, and ear canal for redness, irritation, rash, or drainage
      d. Administer ear drops at room temperature to prevent client discomfort

G. Suppository administration
  1. General information
      a. Is a safe, alternative method of medication administration
      b. Is usually supplied as a solid cone- or oval-shaped mass of medication dissolved in a waxlike substance; body heat melts the wax and releases the medication to be absorbed
      c. Is administered to provide a local or systemic effect
  2. Types
      a. A *rectal suppository* is used when the client is nauseated or vomiting or the medication has an objectionable odor or taste when given orally; this route does not irritate the upper GI tract
      b. A *vaginal suppository* is used to deliver medication directly when treating vaginal infections or inflammation
  3. Purpose
      a. To provide an alternative route of administration
      b. To promote bowel elimination
      c. To treat vaginal infection, pain, or itching
  4. Procedure: Inserting a rectal suppository
      a. Assemble supplies: prescribed suppository, clean disposable gloves, paper towel, and lubricant
      b. Help the client to a left lateral position
      c. Unwrap the suppository and place it on the wrapper
      d. Wash hands and don gloves
      e. Lubricate the smooth, rounded end of the suppository and the gloved index finger
      f. Gently insert the suppository's rounded end into the anus: approximately 4″ (10 cm) for an adult or 2″ (5 cm) or less for a child
      g. With the gloved finger, place the suppository along the rectum wall, and withdraw the finger
      h. Remove gloves by turning them inside out
      i. Press the client's buttocks together for a few seconds
      j. Instruct the client to retain the suppository as long as possible
      k. Wash hands
      l. Assess the client for effects of the medication
  5. Procedure: Inserting a vaginal suppository
      a. Follow the procedure for rectal suppository administration
      b. Help the client to a dorsal recumbent position or a left lateral position

    c. Insert the suppository into the vaginal canal at least 2″ (5 cm)
    d. Instruct the client to lie quietly for 15 minutes
    e. Assess the client for effects of the medication
    f. Wash hands
6. Documentation
    a. Record the drug name, route, dose, method, time administered, initials of nurse administering the drug, and the nurse's signature
    b. Chart the drug's effects
    c. Document the characteristics of any drainage
7. Nursing considerations
    a. Depending on the intended effect of a rectal suppository, determine when the client last had a bowel movement
    b. Give suppositories with an intended systemic effect when the rectum is free of feces, because fecal matter hinders absorption
    c. Before giving a vaginal suppository, clean the perineum with soap and warm water if contaminated with vaginal or rectal secretions

Points to Remember

The five "rights" of medication administration are the right drug, right dose, right client, right route, and right time.

The nurse must use correct medication administration procedures and be knowledgeable about the drug — for the client's safety and the nurse's legal protection.

Before removing a controlled substance from its container in the locked cupboard, the nurse must count the number of units of the drug and check the accuracy of the count.

Before administering any medication, the nurse should discuss the drug and its actions with the client and answer any questions.

Glossary

Enteric — coated to prevent a pill or tablet from being changed by gastric secretions

Meniscus — crescent shape of fluid located at the interface between a liquid and air

Onset of action — interval from drug administration to the start of the drug's effects on body tissues

Ophthalmic — for use in the eye

Otic — for use in the ear

Reconstitution — addition of a diluent to a powdered drug to form an injectable solution

Side effects — unintended or secondary effects of a drug

Therapeutic effect — desired effect of a drug

Administering I.V. Therapy

Learning Objectives

After studying this section, the reader should be able to:

• Describe the three types of I.V. solutions.

• State the purpose of I.V. therapy.

• Review the procedure for starting an I.V. infusion and regulating I.V. flow rate.

• Discuss three methods of I.V. medication administration.

• List the three types of transfusion reactions.

• Describe signs of severe and mild transfusion reactions.

IX. Administering I.V. Therapy

A. Introduction

1. Intravenous (I.V.) therapy is the aseptic instillation of fluids, electrolytes, nutrients, or medications through a needle into a vein
   a. The most common type of I.V. solution contains water plus an additive, such as a nutrient or electrolyte
   b. Electrolyte solutions contain sodium chloride (saline) or dextrose, with water as a base
2. I.V. solutions are isotonic, hypotonic, or hypertonic; the type of solution ordered depends on the client's electrolyte balance
   a. *Isotonic* solutions have the same solute concentration as body fluids and provide fluid volume but do not alter fluid or electrolyte concentration; normal saline (0.9% sodium chloride in water) is an isotonic solution commonly used as initial therapy for dehydration
   b. *Hypotonic* solutions have a solute concentration lower than that normally found in body fluids
   c. *Hypertonic* solutions have a solute concentration higher than that normally found in body fluids
3. I.V. solutions can be given continuously or intermittently
4. Intermittent I.V. fluids or medications can be administered:
   a. Directly into a vein by venipuncture
   b. Via a secondary I.V. line attached to the primary line
   c. Through an injection port of the primary I.V. line
   d. Through an intermittent infusion set (male adapter plug or heparin lock) when an I.V. infusion is not running
5. The I.V. route is used to administer medication when a rapid effect is needed or the medication is too irritating to be given by another route
6. Because an I.V. drug directly enters the bloodstream, it must be infused slowly to prevent severe reactions
7. Problems associated with I.V. administration include infection, fluid infiltration, phlebitis, circulatory overload, and blockage of the infusion
8. Sterile technique is used for all aspects of I.V. therapy to prevent infection; gloves are worn because of possible contact with body fluids
9. Basic equipment for delivering I.V. fluids into a vein includes a bag or bottle for the solution, a needle or similar device to insert the solution into the vein, and connective tubing to deliver the solution to the point of insertion
10. Devices inserted into a vein for instilling I.V. fluids include a winged infusion set (butterfly needle), an inside-the-needle catheter, and an over-the-needle catheter (see *Intravenous insertion devices,* page 110)

B. I.V. fluid infusion

1. General information
   a. The physician orders the amount and type of I.V. solution and any additives (medications or vitamins), specifies the infusion rate, and orders discontinuance of the infusion

INTRAVENOUS INSERTION DEVICES

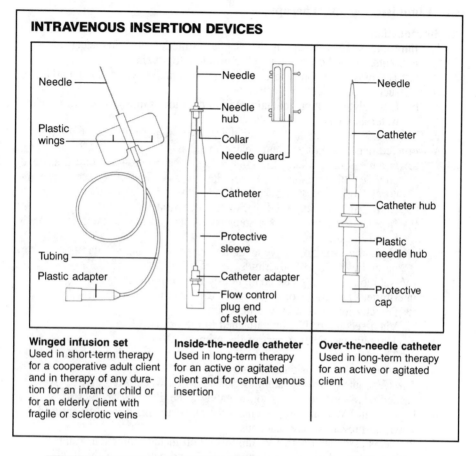

Winged infusion set	Inside-the-needle catheter	Over-the-needle catheter
Used in short-term therapy for a cooperative adult client and in therapy of any duration for an infant or child or for an elderly client with fragile or sclerotic veins	Used in long-term therapy for an active or agitated client and for central venous insertion	Used in long-term therapy for an active or agitated client

    b. The nurse starts, maintains, monitors, and discontinues the infusion
    c. Electronic pumps and controllers are used to maintain the prescribed flow rate
    d. Pumps deliver a preselected volume by adding pressure to the system; controllers use gravity to maintain flow rate; most pumps and controllers can signal problems, such as air in the line or a failing battery
    e. A keep-vein-open rate is just fast enough to keep the vein patent
    f. Institutions usually require hourly assessment of an I.V. infusion, including volume infused, flow rate, and condition of the infusion site
  2. Purpose
    a. To maintain or restore fluid and electrolyte balance
    b. To provide a route for administration of medication or blood for rapid absorption

3. Procedure: Starting an I.V. infusion
   a. Read the physician's order for the amount and type of solution to use and the infusion rate to set
   b. Assemble equipment: prescribed I.V. solution; administration set, including insertion spike, sterile tubing, drip chamber, roller clamp, rubber injection ports, and protective covers for needle adapter and insertion spike; package information, including amount of fluid delivered by drip chamber, either macrodrip (10, 15, or 20 drops/ml of solution) or microdrip (60 drops/ml of solution); I.V. needle or catheter; I.V. pole (free-standing, attached to the bed, or suspended from the ceiling); and padded arm board
   c. Gather supplies: povidone-iodine (Betadine) swabs, alcohol swabs, plastic or paper tape, sterile 2″ × 2″ gauze squares, tourniquet, and clean disposable gloves
   d. Obtain additional supplies, as needed: secondary administration set and solution, volume-control set for children, extension tubing to lengthen original tubing or provide extra injection ports, and I.V. line filter, if not built into the equipment
   e. Wash hands; remove tubing from package and clamp tubing; if solution is in a bag, remove the outer cover (bag may be wet from condensation)
   f. Remove the protective cover from the insertion spike, and remove the protective cap from the I.V. container
   g. Push the insertion spike through the appropriate port on the fluid bag or bottle; hang the bag or bottle; squeeze, then release, the drip chamber until it is half full of fluid
   h. Open the tubing control clamp and clear the tubing of air over an emesis basin or sink; reclamp the tubing
   i. Invert and tap Y injection sites to expel air
   j. Replace the sterile protective cap over the end of the tubing, or attach a covered needle for insertion into the vein
   k. Check the client's identification bracelet
   l. Select an I.V. site; puncture the distal end of the vein first; the most commonly used veins are located from the antecubital space to the wrist (see *Venipuncture sites,* page 112)
   m. Apply a tourniquet above the intended I.V. site; lightly pat the vein if it is not palpable; the vein should feel full, bouncy, and rubbery
   n. Clean the skin thoroughly with povidone-iodine or alcohol swabs, using a circular motion, and allow the skin to dry
   o. Don gloves, and remove the sterile cover from the I.V. needle
   p. Anchor the vein by placing the thumb below it and gently pulling the skin down; insert the needle at a 45-degree angle
   q. Lower the needle after it enters the skin and insert it into the vein either from above or from the side; check for return of blood into the tubing to ensure that the needle is in the vein; carefully advance the needle ½″ to ¾″ (1 to 2 cm)

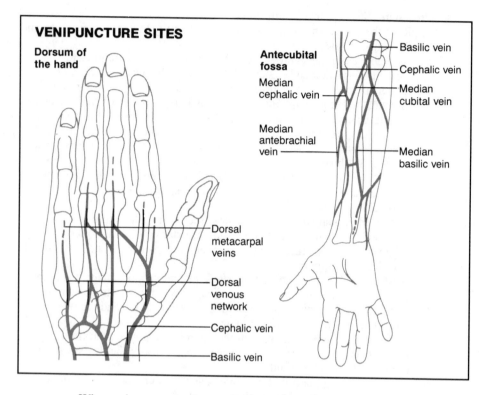

VENIPUNCTURE SITES

Dorsum of the hand

Dorsal metacarpal veins

Dorsal venous network

Cephalic vein

Basilic vein

Antecubital fossa

Median cephalic vein

Median antebrachial vein

Basilic vein

Cephalic vein

Median cubital vein

Median basilic vein

r. When using an over-the-needle catheter, insert the needle and catheter as a unit into the vein, hold the needle hub, and gently advance the plastic catheter over the needle and up the vein to the desired length; do not reinsert the needle; gently withdraw the needle from the catheter with one hand, placing a finger firmly over the catheter

s. When using an inside-the-needle catheter, after inserting the needle and catheter into the vein, thread the catheter through the needle into the vein while holding the catheter in place with finger pressure; withdraw the stylet; never reinsert the stylet

t. Connect the I.V. tubing to the catheter or needle

u. Open the clamp and check the drip chamber for flow of fluids and the I.V. site for swelling

v. Cover the needle with a dressing according to institution policy, and tape it to the client's arm; support the needle by placing a small gauze square or cotton ball under its hub

w. Tape the tubing to the client

x. Set the drip rate as ordered; mark the expected hourly flow rate with tape or a prepared commercial label attached to the I.V. bottle or bag

CALCULATING FLOW RATES

To prevent circulatory overload, the nurse must administer I.V. medication at the prescribed flow rate—the amount of fluid given over a specified time. Use this two-step process to calculate the correct flow rate:

1. Determine the number of milliliters of solution to administer in 1 hour: divide the total amount of solution by the number of hours intended for the infusion.

2. Determine the number of drops of solution to administer in 1 minute—that is, multiply the result in Step 1 by the drop factor of the administration set; then divide by 60.

Calculations for Steps 1 and 2 are combined in the formula below:

$$\frac{\text{Amount of solution} \times \text{drop factor}}{\text{Number of hours to infuse} \times 60 \text{ minutes}} = \text{Flow rate (drops/minute)}$$

y. Write the date, catheter size, and nurse's initials on a piece of tape attached to the dressings; attach a piece of tape with initials and the date on the tubing

z. Remove gloves, dispose of supplies properly, and wash hands

4. Procedure: Monitoring an I.V. infusion

a. Review the physician's order for the amount of solution to be administered and the infusion time prescribed

b. Determine the flow rate by checking the I.V. tubing for its drop factor—the number of drops equivalent to 1 ml; for example, macrodrip tubing can deliver 10, 15, or 20 drops to equal 1 ml; microdrip tubing delivers 60 drops to equal 1 ml (see *Calculating flow rates*)

c. Check the time tape on the bag or bottle to determine the fluid volume remaining

d. Recalculate the flow rate based on this amount

e. Count drops per minute in the drip chamber, and adjust the drip rate if necessary

f. Ensure that the infusion rate and other controls on the pump or controller are correctly set and that the pump or controller is operating according to the manufacturer's guidelines

g. Assess the I.V. site, drip rate, volume infused, and correct operation of the device at least every hour

5. Procedure: Discontinuing infusion

a. Gather equipment: clean disposable gloves, alcohol or povidone-iodine swab, sterile dressing

b. Wash hands

c. Clamp the I.V. tubing with roller clamp

d. Loosen the tape without dislodging the needle

e. Don gloves and hold an alcohol or povidone-iodine swab over the I.V. site

f. Withdraw the needle or catheter

g. Apply firm pressure to the site with the swab for 2 to 3 minutes
h. Check the needle or catheter for damage; report a broken device to the charge nurse immediately
i. Apply a sterile dressing
j. Discard used supplies in an appropriate receptacle; remove gloves and wash hands

6. Documentation
   a. Document insertion time and site, type of device used, flow rate, type and amount of infusion fluid, and nurse's initials and signature
   b. Note the condition of the I.V. site
   c. Chart hourly or according to institution policy the amount of fluid infused on the intake and output sheet or special I.V. administration record

7. Nursing considerations
   a. Know institution policy regarding I.V. infusion
   b. Check the solution before administration, according to the five "rights" of safe drug administration (see Section VIII); ensure that additives are in the solution and that the I.V. bag or bottle is labeled with the names and doses of additives; check the solution for color, clarity, and expiration date
   c. Open all supplies using sterile technique; during the infusion, maintain sterility of parts of the administration set and supplies that are inside the I.V. system (such as insertion spikes) or are inserted into the skin (such as needles or catheters)
   d. If difficulties arise in trying to distend the vein, apply a warm washcloth to the area, ask the client to open and close a fist, or lower the arm below heart level
   e. Apply a dressing over the I.V. site according to institution policy; some institutions require that an antiseptic ointment, such as povidone-iodine, be applied before using a small gauze dressing; others require a transparent occlusive dressing through which the site can be observed
   f. Assess the I.V. site every hour, and report signs of inflammation or infiltration
   g. Change the I.V. site every 48 to 72 hours and all tubing every 24 to 48 hours; use administration sets for blood, blood products, and lipids once, then discard them
   h. Because equipment may vary, carefully follow manufacturer's instructions for use
   i. If the alarm sounds on the controller or pump, ensure that fluid remains in the bag or bottle, the tubing is not pinched or kinked, the tubing clamp is completely open, the I.V. line is not infiltrated, the drip chamber is correctly filled, and the drop sensor and I.V. container are correctly placed

C. I.V. medication administration

1. General information
   a. I.V. medication is injected with a needle or through tubing directly into a vein, producing a systemic effect within seconds
   b. A *primary I.V. line* consists of the I.V. bag or bottle and the tubing through which the solution flows
   c. A *piggyback* is a smaller I.V. bag or bottle usually containing medication in a solution and connected to the primary I.V. line tubing at the upper port
   d. A *secondary set* is a second container connected to the primary I.V. line at the lower port
   e. A *volume control set* (Soluset, Volutrol, Buretrol) — a container attached below the primary I.V. bag or bottle — can be intermittently filled with a measured volume of fluid and closed off from the bag or bottle by a roller closure device; commonly used for pediatric clients or when fluid volume must be carefully measured and controlled
   f. An *I.V. bolus* (or I.V. push) is a mass or pulse of fluid or medication administered as a single dose as rapidly as possible, usually through an I.V. tubing port or heparin lock
   g. A *heparin lock* (or heparin well) is a venous access device intermittently filled with heparin or saline solution to prevent clotting between injections of fluid or medication
2. Purpose
   a. To achieve immediate systemic effects from a medication
   b. To provide the client with medication too irritating to tissues if given by other routes
   c. To maintain therapeutic blood levels of a drug, such as an antibiotic
3. Procedure: Administering a drug with a primary I.V. bag or bottle
   a. Assemble equipment and supplies: correct sterile medication and diluent, if required, antiseptic swabs (povidone-iodine or alcohol), sterile syringe of appropriate size, 1″ to 1½″ (2.5 to 3.8 cm) needle, and medication label
   b. Check the physician's order carefully for the drug name, dosage, and route
   c. Confirm the compatibility of the drug and solution being mixed
   d. Prepare medication from an ampule or vial (use a filter needle if mandated by institution policy)
   e. Locate the injection port on the I.V. fluid container, and clean it with an antiseptic swab
   f. Close the I.V. flow clamp; insert the syringe needle through the port and inject the medication
   g. Attach a medication label to the I.V. container
   h. Rotate the container to mix the medication and solution
   i. Open the flow clamp and regulate the flow rate

4. Procedure: Administering a drug with a piggyback or secondary set
   a. Check the piggyback or secondary set for medication; if necessary, add the drug, using the same procedure as for a primary I.V. bag or bottle
   b. Insert the spike of the administration set into a secondary bottle or bag, and attach a 1″ (2.5 cm) needle to the I.V. tubing (some administration sets have a preattached needle)
   c. Label the tubing with the date, time, and nurse's signature
   d. Clean the injection port of the primary line's tubing with an antiseptic swab; insert the needle into the port (lower port for piggyback; upper port for secondary set)
   e. Regulate the flow rate to infuse over 30 to 60 minutes (the primary infusion begins when the secondary container is empty)
   f. Secure the needle in the port with tape.
   g. Position the primary I.V. bottle or bag at the same level as a secondary container or lower than a piggyback
   h. When the infusion is complete, readjust the flow rate
5. Procedure: Administering a drug with a volume control set
   a. Add 50 to 100 ml of fluid from the primary I.V. bottle or bag to the volume control administration set
   b. Shut off inflow to the fluid chamber by closing the roller clamp above the volume control chamber
   c. Clean the injection port with an antiseptic swab; insert the syringe needle into the port and inject the medication
   d. Rotate the fluid chamber to mix the medication
   e. Regulate the flow rate with the roller clamp below the fluid chamber
   f. Attach a medication label to the fluid chamber
6. Procedure: Administering a drug with an I.V. bolus
   a. Prepare medication in the syringe
   b. Check the compatibility of the medication with the I.V. solution
   c. Clean the injection port of the I.V. tubing with an antiseptic swab
   d. Pinch the tubing above the port, insert the needle, draw back on the plunger to withdraw blood, and unpinch the tubing
   e. Inject the medication at the specified rate, and withdraw the needle
7. Procedure: Administering a drug with a heparin lock
   a. Prepare two syringes with normal saline solution and one syringe with 0.5 ml of 100 units/ml heparin, or use prefilled syringes; label the syringes; prepare syringe or piggyback infusion set with the prescribed medication
   b. Clean the injection port of the heparin lock; insert the needle of a syringe prepared with normal saline solution, withdrawing blood to ensure that the needle is in the vein
   c. Inject 2 ml of normal saline solution and remove the syringe
   d. Insert the needle of the syringe or piggyback infusion set with the prescribed medication into the heparin lock
   e. Slowly inject the prescribed medication at the recommended rate, or adjust the flow rate of the piggyback set

    f. When the injection or infusion is complete, withdraw the needle and inject the recommended amount of saline solution, using the second normal saline syringe

    g. Insert the heparin syringe, and flush heparin slowly into the heparin lock

8. Documentation

    a. Record the drug name, dose, time administered, route, site, and nurse's initials and signature; I.V. medication is usually recorded on the medication administration record or nurses' notes and on the I.V. flow sheet

    b. Assess the client's response to the medication, and document any therapeutic effects or side effects in the nurses' notes

9. Nursing considerations

    a. Know institution policy regarding who is permitted to administer I.V. medication

    b. Check the compatibility of the medication with the primary solution; an additional injection site may be necessary if medication is incompatible

    c. Before injecting I.V. medication, withdraw blood to ensure that the needle or catheter is in the vein

    d. Always label the I.V. bag or bottle and tubing, especially when adding a new container, changing tubing, or injecting medication into the I.V. container

    e. Assess the I.V. site frequently for swelling, redness, and tenderness

    f. Assess patency of the heparin lock at least every 8 hours by aspirating blood; flush with 2 ml of normal saline solution, and refill with new heparin solution

    g. Check institution policy on flushing the heparin lock; some institutions recommend using normal saline alone to maintain patency of an intermittent I.V. device

D. Blood transfusion

1. General information

    a. During a blood transfusion, whole blood or its components are introduced into a vein

    b. The procedure is indicated in clients who have had massive blood loss, such as in hypovolemic shock, or who require replacement of blood volume or blood components lost in surgery, childbirth, trauma, or a disease, such as leukemia

    c. Blood transfusions must be matched to the client's blood type (A, B, O, AB), Rh group, and other factors; the test used to match blood factors is called *typing and crossmatching*

    d. Blood transfusions are administered through a secondary set connected to a primary I.V. line that contains only normal saline solution; normal saline is isotonic and reduces hemolysis (rupture) of red blood cells, whereas dextrose 5% in water causes hemolysis, and lactated Ringer's solution causes blood clotting

    e. The procedure requires two health care professionals (some institutions require two registered nurses) to verify the client's name, identification number, blood type, and Rh group; the blood bag's expiration date; and the product unit numbers

2. Transfusion reactions
   a. *Hemolytic* transfusion reactions are antigen-antibody responses caused by a mismatched blood type or Rh factor and produce hemolysis of red blood cells
   b. *Allergic* reactions may result from a substance in the donor's blood, which is recognized as an antigen when introduced into the client's body
   c. *Febrile* (bacterial) reactions, caused by contaminated blood, occur rarely
3. Purpose
   a. To replace blood volume or blood components lost during surgery or through injury or disease
   b. To maintain circulating blood volume
4. Procedure: Administering a blood transfusion
   a. Obtain baseline data of the client's blood pressure, pulse, temperature, respirations, known allergies, and blood study results
   b. Ensure that the consent form (if required) is signed
   c. Assemble supplies and equipment: 18G or larger needle, normal saline solution, Y set for blood transfusion with appropriate blood filter, clean disposable gloves, and other supplies as needed, such as equipment for starting an I.V. line
   d. Obtain the units of blood to be infused from the laboratory; check the client's name, identification number, blood type, and Rh group; the blood donor number; and the blood's expiration date (verify it with the laboratory technician); sign the appropriate form
   e. Have another nurse compare information on the laboratory blood type record with the name and identification number on the client's bracelet and with the number and identifying information on the blood bag label; sign appropriate forms with the other nurse
   f. Wash hands and don gloves
   g. Gently invert the blood bag several times to mix blood and plasma
   h. Set both roller clamps to the "off" position; insert one spike in the blood bag and one in the bottle or bag of normal saline solution; prime the tubing with normal saline
   i. Attach primed tubing to the I.V. needle and tape it securely; open the saline and main roller clamps to establish the I.V. flow
   j. Close the saline and main roller clamps; squeeze the blood drip chamber until the filter is covered with blood; open the main roller clamp and regulate blood flow so that a unit of blood is infused over 1½ to 2 hours

    k. Regulate blood flow for 15 minutes at 20 drops/minute; stay with the client for at least 15 minutes, taking vital signs every 5 minutes; observe the client for signs of a transfusion reaction (sudden chills, nausea, vomiting, rash, and tachycardia); if a transfusion reaction occurs, clamp the blood tubing, open the normal saline line, and notify the charge nurse

    l. If no reaction occurs, adjust the flow rate as ordered

    m. Assess vital signs after 15 minutes, then every 30 minutes until the transfusion is completed; tell the client to call a nurse if any unusual feelings or itching, swelling, chest pain, or dyspnea occurs

    n. After blood is infused, clamp the blood flow and open the normal saline clamp to clear the blood line with normal saline

    o. On the form attached to the blood unit, record the time of infusion and amount of blood infused; return one copy to the blood bank with the blood bag, and place a second copy in the client's chart

5. Documentation

    a. Record the start and completion time of the transfusion, the amount of blood given, and the blood unit number

    b. Chart vital signs and assessment data during the transfusion

    c. Document signs of transfusion reaction (such as tachycardia, fever, flank pain, dyspnea, and chills) and nursing actions in response to reactions

6. Nursing considerations

    a. Confirm that the physician's order has been issued and that a consent form has been signed before starting a blood transfusion

    b. Keep normal saline solution infusing until the transfusion is completed to flush the line of blood and to keep it open for supportive measures if a transfusion reaction occurs

    c. Start a transfusion within 30 minutes after the blood arrives at the bedside or is removed from refrigeration

    d. Wear gloves when starting or discontinuing a transfusion, disposing of a blood bag and equipment, or performing any procedure that may contaminate hands with the client's blood to prevent transfer of blood-borne diseases, such as hepatitis and acquired immunodeficiency syndrome

    e. Check the client carefully for transfusion reactions: signs of acute reaction include sudden chills, fever, headache, low back pain, chest pain, drop in blood pressure, nausea, flushing, agitation, severe dyspnea, and bronchospasm; signs of less severe reaction include hives and itching but no fever

Points to Remember

Because I.V. fluids and medications are administered directly into the venous circulation, they must be prepared and administered carefully and accurately.

Some institutions allow only physicians or specially prepared nurses to administer medication by I.V. bolus.

To prevent contamination, the nurse must wear gloves when handling supplies and equipment or when performing certain procedures (such as discontinuing an I.V. infusion).

The nurse must always label the I.V. bag or bottle and tubing, especially when adding a new container, changing tubing, or injecting medication into an I.V. container.

Glossary

Circulatory overload — condition in which the intravascular fluid compartment contains more fluid than normal, usually the result of too rapid administration of I.V. fluids; can lead to pulmonary edema and heart failure

Flow rate — number of drops of solution given in 1 minute or milliliters administered in 1 hour

Infiltration — deposit or diffusion into tissue of a substance, usually fluid, not normally found there; infiltration of I.V. fluids results when a needle or catheter is incorrectly placed outside a vein and causes skin swelling

I.V. bolus — mass or pulse of fluid or medication administered as rapidly as possible

Phlebitis — inflammation of a vein caused by trauma or chemical irritation and manifested by redness, warmth, pain, and swelling

Providing Wound Care

Learning Objectives

After studying this section, the reader should be able to:

● Describe the procedure for applying a dry sterile dressing.

● Discuss nursing actions for shortening a drain, emptying a closed drainage system, removing sutures and staples, and irrigating a wound.

● Cite the purpose of each wound care procedure.

● Describe information that the nurse must document after performing wound care.

● Differentiate between dry sterile and wet-to-dry dressings.

● Identify the purpose of bandages and binders and describe the proper application of each.

X. Providing Wound Care

A. Introduction

1. A wound, usually associated with a break in skin integrity, can be caused intentionally (as in surgery) or accidentally (as in trauma)
2. Wounds heal by primary or secondary intention
   a. Healing by *primary intention* occurs when wound edges are approximated (close together) and little tissue is lost
   b. Healing by *secondary intention* occurs when wound edges are not approximated and some tissue is lost, as in a pressure ulcer
   c. Wounds healing by secondary intention are left open until they fill with scar tissue; such wounds take longer to heal, leave more scarring, and are more likely to become infected
3. Risk factors that can delay wound healing include malnutrition, obesity, anti-inflammatory or immunosuppressive drugs, smoking, and certain diseases, such as diabetes mellitus
4. Delayed wound healing can lead to infection
   a. Clinical signs of infection begin 36 to 48 hours after surgery or trauma
   b. Signs of wound infection include increased temperature, pulse rate, and respiratory rate; progressive edema and wound tenderness; and redness of wound edges (unless infection is in deeper tissues)
5. Wounds are cared for by open (no dressings cover the wound) or closed (dressings cover the wound) methods
6. A nurse is responsible for:
   a. Assessing the dressing or wound
   b. Implementing wound care orders written by a physician
   c. Changing dressings
   d. Preventing infection by using sterile technique when providing wound care

B. Dry sterile dressing application

1. General information
   a. Is a wound covering, usually made of absorbent material (such as gauze) but can also be made of nonadhering material (Telfa), transparent self-adhesive film (Tegaderm), or hydrocolloid occlusive material (Op-site)
   b. Has three layers—the first layer covers the wound and collects blood, fibrin, and debris; the second layer collects excess drainage; the outer layer protects the wound from external contamination
   c. The physician changes the initial dressing after surgery, then orders dressing changes daily or as needed
   d. Changing a dressing involves assessing the wound, protecting it from infection, and possibly cleaning or irrigating the wound
   e. Wound assessment entails observing the wound for signs of healing and approximation (closing) of wound edges, drainage, edema, odor, and client complaints of pain or tenderness

    f. Agents commonly used to clean wounds include povidone-iodine (Betadine) solution, 70% alcohol, 3% hydrogen peroxide, and sterile normal saline solution

2. Purpose
   a. To promote wound healing
   b. To absorb blood and drainage from the wound
   c. To prevent pathogens from entering the wound
   d. To remove drainage, blood, debris, and harmful microorganisms from the wound

3. Procedure: Applying a dry sterile dressing
   a. Read the physician's order to determine when the dressing must be changed and any specific orders, such as the physician's protocol for cleaning the wound
   b. Read the nursing care plan or interview the client about personal preferences, if choices are permitted
   c. Discuss the dressing change with the client, including an explanation of how the client can participate and how to protect sterile supplies from contamination
   d. Assemble supplies: clean disposable gloves; sterile gloves; plastic bag for soiled dressings; tape; mask (if required by the institution); sterile dressing change tray or supplies from a central supply cart, including sterile drape or towel, gauze dressings, large outer dressing (Surgipad or abdominal pad), bath blanket, and waterproof pad
   e. Gather additional supplies as needed: cleansing solution, cotton balls, gauze or large applicators to clean the wound, container for cleansing solution, sterile forceps, sterile normal saline solution, ointment, and sterile tongue blade to apply ointment
   f. Place the client in a comfortable position; expose the wound only, using a bath blanket if necessary
   g. Tape a cuffed, open plastic bag to the bedside table
   h. Loosen the tape of the old dressing by holding down the skin and pulling the tape gently but firmly toward the wound
   i. Wash hands, and don clean gloves and mask, if necessary
   j. Carefully remove soiled dressing; if the inner dressing adheres to the wound or drain, moisten with a small amount of sterile normal saline solution; remove the inner dressing with sterile forceps, taking care not to dislodge any drains
   k. Assess the amount, type, and odor of drainage; assess the wound for healing, approximation of wound edges, edema, dehiscence (wound gaping), and painfulness
   l. Discard the dressing in a plastic bag without touching the outside of the bag; remove gloves and place in the plastic bag; wash hands
   m. Open the dressing change tray or sterile supplies using sterile technique; pour sterile cleansing solution over sterile gauze sponges in a sterile container, and don sterile gloves

n. Clean the wound using a separate swab moistened with solution for each stroke; clean from the least to the most contaminated area; clean from top to bottom or from the center outward; clean the area around the drain, moving from the center outward in a circular motion after the wound is cleaned; dry the wound with gauze squares, using the same motions (see *Cleaning a wound*)

o. If ordered, apply ointment or medication to the wound, using a sterile applicator or tongue blade

p. Apply sterile dressings to the wound one at a time, using a sterile gloved hand or tissue forceps; place sterile gauze under and around the drain

q. Apply the large outer dressing, touching only the outside, typically marked by a colored line down the middle; the outer dressing can be applied with an ungloved hand

r. Remove gloves from the inside out, and discard them in a plastic bag

s. Secure the dressing with tape, a binder, or tie tapes, such as Montgomery straps, if frequent changing is required

t. Wash hands, remove all supplies, and help the client to a comfortable position

4. Documentation
   a. Document wound assessment, including the wound's appearance and the color, amount, and odor of drainage
   b. Record the type of solution used and the type of dressing applied
   c. Chart the client's tolerance of the procedure

5. Nursing considerations
   a. Check institution policy and procedure; some institutions have special carts containing dressings and supplies for wound care that can be wheeled to the client's room for dressing changes
   b. Use paper or hypoallergenic tape for a client who is allergic to tape or whose skin is thin and fragile
   c. Apply transparent air-occlusive dressings (such as Op-site) directly over a small wound
   d. Reinforce a dressing saturated with blood, check the client's vital signs, and notify the charge nurse
   e. Assess the dressing over a new wound every 15 to 30 minutes during the first few hours to detect signs of hemorrhage; after the client becomes stable, check the dressing or wound at least once per shift
   f. Replace any dressing that becomes wet from the outside — such as from a spilled drink, bath water, or urine — as soon as possible to prevent wound contamination

C. Penrose drain care

1. General information
   a. A drain is a hollow tube through which secretions are removed from the wound cavity

CLEANING A WOUND

These illustrations show how to maintain asepsis when cleaning a wound. Numbers and arrows indicate the appropriate sequence and direction to follow when moving the swab, always progressing from clean (top or center of wound) to unclean (bottom or outer) areas.

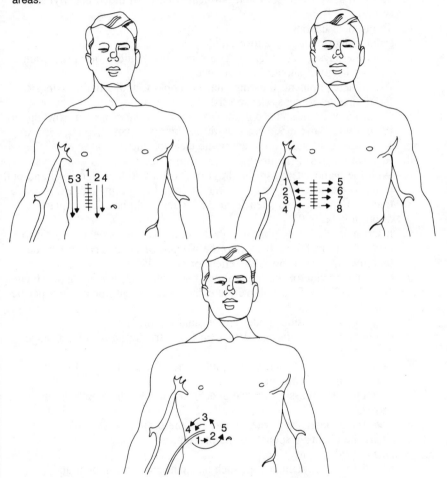

b. A Penrose drain is a flexible rubber tube inserted through an incision or through a separate opening made a few centimeters away from an incision; it is an "open" drain because it collects exudate onto an absorbent gauze dressing

c. Without a drain, some wounds heal on the surface while drainage collects inside, interfering with healing and risking abscess formation

d. Because wounds heal from the inside to the outside, a physician may order that the drain be pulled out, or shortened, 1″ to 2″ (2.5 to 5 cm) every day to facilitate drainage and healing; in some institutions, this procedure is performed only by a physician

2. Purpose
   a. To drain serosanguineous and purulent fluid from tissue underlying the wound
   b. To promote healing
3. Procedure: Shortening a Penrose drain
   a. Read the physician's order to determine who should shorten the drain and the length it should be shortened
   b. Assemble equipment: dressing change supplies, additional dressings for the drain site, forceps, sterile scissors, sterile safety pin, and hemostat
   c. Clean the skin around the drain site using a circular motion, starting at the drain site and moving outward; use one swab for each stroke; use forceps to hold the drain erect while cleaning the skin around it
   d. Remove sutures if the drain is sutured in place
   e. With the hemostat, grasp the drain by its full width at skin level and pull it out to the specified length (if the drain is being removed, exert gentle traction until it is extracted from the wound and place it in a plastic disposable bag)
   f. Insert a sterile safety pin through the drain as it exits near the skin to prevent it from falling back into the wound; be careful not to pull the drain out further or prick the client or yourself
   g. Cut off a portion of the drain above the safety pin, leaving approximately 1″ to 2 ″ (2.5 to 5 cm) above the skin; place the cut portion in a plastic bag
   h. Apply gauze dressings under and around the drain
   i. Continue the procedure as described for a dry sterile dressing change
4. Documentation
   a. Record the amount, color, odor, and other characteristics of drainage found on the old dressings
   b. Document the dressing change and, if applicable, the length the drain was shortened
   c. Note the appearance of the wound and the drain insertion site
   d. Chart the client's response to the procedure
5. Nursing considerations
   a. Check for signs of infection, such as changes in the amount and characteristics of drainage and an increase in body temperature
   b. Be careful not to remove the drain when removing the dressing or cleaning the drain site
   c. When changing the dressing, inspect the wound and identify the type of drain, its location, and whether it is sutured in place
   d. Examine the skin around the drain for excoriation, inflammation, or rash

D. Closed wound drainage system maintenance
1. General information
   a. A closed wound drainage system is used to promote healing by applying suction to surgical wounds that contain large amounts of drainage
   b. Draining helps to reduce the risk of infection and skin breakdown and to decrease the number of dressing changes needed
   c. The system consists of perforated tubing connected to a portable vacuum device; tubing lies within the wound and usually exits the body from a site near the primary suture line to preserve wound integrity
   d. The drainage tubing is inserted during surgery, sutured loosely in place, and removed when the wound is free of drainage
   e. The vacuum withdraws drainage from the wound into a closed collection container; gentle, even pressure is exerted on tissues when the collection reservoir is compressed manually
2. Purpose
   a. To suction excessive drainage from a surgical wound
   b. To promote wound healing and prevent infection
3. Procedure: Emptying a closed wound drainage system
   a. Assemble supplies: clean disposable gloves, clean graduated container, and sterile container, if specimen must be obtained
   b. Wash hands and don gloves
   c. Place the clean graduated container next to the collection reservoir; locate and open the drainage plug
   d. Invert the collection reservoir and empty it into the graduated container (if a specimen must be collected, empty a drainage sample into the sterile container; then empty the remaining drainage into the graduated container)
   e. Reestablish suction by squeezing the reservoir flat; maintain suction by closing the drainage plug
   f. Measure the amount of drainage (see *Maintaining a closed wound drainage system,* page 128)
4. Documentation
   a. Document the procedure and the amount and characteristics of drainage
   b. Record whether a specimen is sent to the laboratory and the time it is sent
   c. Note the amount of drainage on the fluid intake and output sheet
5. Nursing considerations
   a. Examine the drainage system regularly to ensure proper functioning
   b. During the first days after surgery, assess characteristics and amount of drainage at least once per shift (more frequently if the client's condition warrants); copious drainage is likely
   c. Empty the collection reservoir to monitor the amount of drainage, to prevent reflux of drainage into the wound, and to maintain proper functioning of the drainage system
   d. Empty the collection reservoir as needed or when drainage reaches the "full" line (at least once per shift)

MAINTAINING A CLOSED WOUND DRAINAGE SYSTEM

A portable wound drainage system draws drainage from the wound site, such as the chest wall after a mastectomy, by means of tubing. To empty drainage, remove the plug and turn the unit up-side down. Al- low drainage to collect in the small graduated container. To reestablish suction, compress the system against a firm surface to expel all the air, and replace the plug.

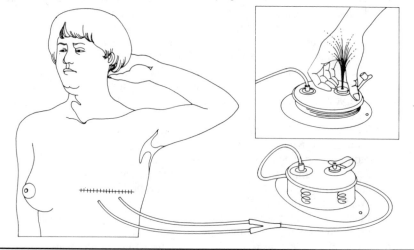

e. Use sterile technique to prevent introduction of pathogens into the wound when handling the wound or emptying the collection reservoir
f. If the client's drainage system has several tubes, label the origin and purpose of each for easy identification
g. Position the collection reservoir below the wound level
h. During client ambulation, pin the collection container to the client's gown

E. Wet-to-dry dressing application
1. General information
   a. Wet-to-dry dressings consist of a moistened dressing packed into or placed on a wound, covered with dry dressings, then allowed to dry
   b. The wet gauze, as it dries, traps necrotic tissue and drainage; when the dressing is removed, the infected and necrotic material is removed with it (debridement)
   c. Wet-to-dry dressings are used on wounds (such as pressure ulcers) or burns that heal by secondary intention
   d. The dressing is moistened with a solution, such as sterile normal saline, 10% povidone-iodine (Betadine), 0.25% acetic acid, 3% hydrogen peroxide, and sodium hypochlorite (Dakin's)
   e. Cotton fibers should not be used because they can pull loose and remain in the wound, encouraging bacterial growth and contamination

      f. Excessively wet dressings that do not dry before the next dressing change can cause maceration or increased risk of bacterial growth

  2. Purpose

      a. To debride large wounds whose edges cannot be approximated

      b. To promote wound healing by secondary intention

      c. To treat wound infections

  3. Procedure: Applying a wet-to-dry dressing

      a. Assemble supplies: clean disposable gloves, sterile disposable gloves, sterile synthetic gauze dressings, sterile basin, sterile solution as ordered by the physician, sterile gloves, sterile forceps, plastic bag, and tape or tie tapes (Montgomery straps)

      b. Pour solution into the sterile basin and don clean gloves

      c. Remove soiled dressings, touching only the gauze; free the inner dressing quickly but do not moisten the dressing to remove it, so the dried exudate and necrotic tissue are removed with the dressing

      d. Assess wound appearance and drainage on the dressing

      e. Discard the dressing in a plastic bag; remove and discard gloves

      f. Wash hands, open the sterile supplies, and don sterile gloves

      g. Place the new dressing into the prepared solution, and wring excess moisture from it

      h. Pack a moistened dressing into the wound, pressing it into all depressions and cracks; use sterile forceps as necessary to insert gauze

      i. Apply a dry dressing; then place a large dressing (abdominal pad or Surgipad) over the wet and dry dressings

      j. Remove gloves and place them in a plastic bag

      k. Secure the dressing by taping its edges or using tie tapes

      l. Discard soiled materials; wash hands

  4. Documentation

      a. Record the type of dressing applied, solution used, and application time

      b. Document the wound's appearance and the amount and characteristics of drainage

  5. Nursing considerations

      a. Use the correct strength of prescribed solution; solutions are prescribed according to wound type

      b. Never place an occlusive covering over a wet-to-dry dressing because it interferes with the drying of the inner dressing

      c. Be prepared to culture the wound if signs of infection develop

F. Suture and staple removal

  1. General information

      a. Sutures are stitches made of silk, cotton, linen, wire, nylon, or Dacron and used to approximate body tissue

      b. Staples are silver or wire clips used to approximate body tissue

      c. Stay or retention sutures are used to attach underlying fat and muscle as well as skin in an obese client or one at risk for poor healing; usually left in place 14 to 21 days

d. Skin sutures are either interrupted (each stitch tied and knotted individually) or continuous (one thread used in a series of stitches and tied at the beginning and end)

e. In some institutions, only physicians remove sutures or staples; other institutions permit nurses to remove skin sutures with a physician's order; generally, only physicians remove stay sutures

f. Sutures are cut next to the skin with sterile scissors and pulled out with forceps

g. Staples are removed with a sterile surgical staple remover that squeezes the center of the staple to remove it from the skin

h. Skin sutures or staples are usually removed 7 to 10 days after surgery or trauma; every other interrupted suture may be removed one day and the remaining sutures 1 to 2 days later

2. Purpose
   a. To prevent a skin reaction to foreign materials
   b. To encourage natural healing of an incision
   c. To prevent wound infection

3. Procedure: Removing sutures or staples
   a. Review the physician's order and institution policy
   b. Discuss suture or staple removal with the client, noting that removal may cause a stinging or pulling sensation; ask the client not to touch the wound
   c. Assemble supplies: suture removal set (includes sterile forceps and scissors) or staple remover, antiseptic swabs, sterile dressing set or sterile dressing supplies, sterile butterfly tape to hold wound edges together if separation occurs, plastic bag, clean disposable gloves, and sterile disposable gloves
   d. Wash hands and don clean gloves
   e. Remove old dressings; discard dressings and gloves in the plastic bag
   f. Wash hands, open the sterile packages, and don sterile gloves
   g. Clean the incision with antiseptic swabs, moving from the least to most contaminated area
   h. To remove sutures, grasp at the knot with forceps
   i. Place the curved tip of suture scissors as close as possible to the skin under the knot; cut the suture
   j. With forceps, pull the suture out in one piece and inspect it to ensure complete removal
   k. To remove staples, place the staple remover under the center of the staple, compress the staple remover, and remove the staple (see *Removing a staple*)
   l. Drop each removed suture or staple into the plastic bag
   m. Clean the incision with an antiseptic solution, and cover it with a dry sterile dressing, if ordered
   n. Remove gloves by turning them inside out and put them in the plastic bag; discard or disinfect used articles

REMOVING A STAPLE

To remove a staple, position the staple remover beneath the staple's span. Squeeze the staple remover's handles until they close completely; then lift the staple as shown.

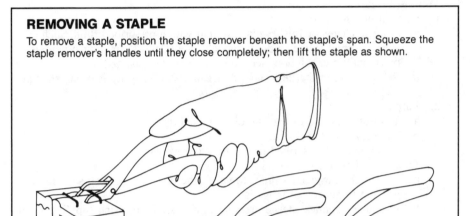

4. Documentation
   a. Document the procedure on the appropriate form
   b. Note the wound's condition and characteristics of any drainage
   c. Record wound cleaning and the type of dressings applied
   d. Document any client teaching related to future wound care
5. Nursing considerations
   a. Review institution policy and procedures for suture or staple removal
   b. Before removing sutures or staples, assess wound healing and check for evidence of infection or dehiscence
   c. If healing is progressing poorly, anticipate removing random or every other suture before removing all sutures
   d. Check for wound separation after removing sutures or staples; if slight separation occurs, apply butterfly tape or adhesive skin closures (Steri-strips) over the gap; if extensive dehiscence occurs, cover the wound with sterile gauze and report it to the charge nurse or physician
   e. Review institution policy on use of adhesive skin closures; some physicians routinely order adhesive skin closures after suture or staple removal
   f. Monitor wound appearance after removing the sutures or staples

G. Wound irrigation

1. General information
   a. A nurse cleans or flushes out a wound with a prescribed fluid, such as sterile normal saline, sodium hypochlorite (Dakin's), hydrogen peroxide, or an antibiotic solution (see *Common irrigating solutions*)
   b. Requires use of sterile technique because skin integrity is diminished at the wound site
2. Purpose
   a. To clean a wound of exudate or tissue debris
   b. To apply heat to a wound
   c. To administer prescribed medication to a wound
3. Procedure: Irrigating a wound
   a. Review the physician's order to verify the type of irrigating solution to use and frequency of irrigation
   b. Assemble supplies: sterile dressing tray or sterile dressing supplies, sterile irrigating syringe (with soft catheter if the wound is deep), sterile basin to hold irrigating solution, sterile irrigating solution (usually 150 to 500 ml of normal saline warmed to 90° F [32° C]), clean basin to collect used irrigating solution, sterile disposable gloves, waterproof pad, clean disposable gloves, and plastic disposable bag
   c. Position the client so the solution flows by gravity from the wound's upper end to the lower end and into the collection basin
   d. Place a waterproof pad under the wound area, and place a plastic bag for disposal of soiled supplies within easy reach
   e. Position the collection basin on the waterproof pad below the wound, as close to the wound as possible without touching it
   f. Wash hands, don clean gloves, remove soiled dressing, and discard gloves and dressing in the plastic bag
   g. Don sterile gloves and prepare a sterile field with irrigating syringe, sterile basin, and dressings
   h. Fill the sterile basin with warmed prescribed solution, and fill the syringe with irrigating solution
   i. Irrigate the wound with a gentle, steady stream of solution, beginning at the wound's upper end; if a catheter is used for a deep wound, attach it to the filled irrigating syringe and insert it into the wound until it meets resistance; then begin irrigating
   j. Continue irrigation until all the prescribed solution is used or the solution runs clear
   k. Dry the area around the wound with sterile gauze, and assess the wound's appearance
   l. Apply dry sterile dressing to the wound
4. Documentation
   a. Record the procedure, the type and amount of solution used, and the color, amount, and odor of the returned solution
   b. Document the wound's appearance and the color, amount, and odor of any exudate

COMMON IRRIGATING SOLUTIONS	
SOLUTION	DESCRIPTION
Acetic acid	Used for draining wounds infected with gram-positive or gram-negative organisms, especially *Pseudomonas;* used as 0.25% solution; can cause excoriation of skin around a wound
Povidone-iodine (Betadine)	Used for draining wounds infected with staphylococcus or aerobic bacteria; a broad-spectrum antiseptic used as 10% solution; can dry and stain the client's skin
Sodium hypochlorite (Dakin's)	Used as an antiseptic to dissolve necrotic tissue; can cause skin breakdown; new solution must be prepared every 24 hours because solution is unstable
Hydrogen peroxide	Used in a half-strength solution; aids mechanical debridement; may alter new tissue formation because of its foaming action
Normal saline	Used for clean wounds because it has no bactericidal properties; aids mechanical debridement
Antibiotic	Contain neomycin (Mycifradin), chloramphenicol (Chloromycetin), gentamicin (Garamycin), or carbenicillin (Geopen); use is controversial because may permit overgrowth of resistant organisms

      c. Note signs of wound healing, inflammation, or infection
      d. Document the client's response to the procedure
   5. Nursing considerations
      a. Assess the client's degree of pain before irrigating the wound; administer an analgesic as ordered 30 to 40 minutes before the procedure, if indicated
      b. If the prescribed irrigating solution may irritate surrounding skin, apply sterile petrolatum to the skin, using a sterile tongue blade
      c. Evaluate the wound for healing or infection

H. Bandage and binder application
   1. General information: Bandages
      a. A bandage is a strip of cloth used to wrap or support a body part or to secure a dressing; a *roller bandage* is a lengthy strip of woven cloth, gauze, or elastic fabric wound onto itself to form a cylinder or roll (see *Bandaging techniques,* pages 134 and 135)
      b. Commonly used bandages are made of gauze, rayon and polyester (Kling), crinoline, flannel, muslin, and elastic materials
      c. Gauze is lightweight and porous and molds to the body; can be soaked with petrolatum or other medication for application to a wound
      d. Kling, a woven rayon-polyester gauze, stretches and molds to the body

BANDAGING TECHNIQUES

When applying a bandage, face the client. Hold a roller bandage in the dominant hand, with the beginning of the roll uppermost; unroll the bandage about 3″ (8 cm) to start. Place a flat bandage surface on the anterior surface of the body part to be covered, and hold the end in place with the thumb of the nondominant hand. Wrap the bandage around the body part with one or more basic turns, using even pressure. Secure the end of the bandage with tape or a metal clip.

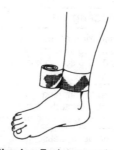

Circular: Each turn encircles the previous turn, completely covering it; used for anchoring a bandage

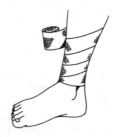

Spiral: Each turn partially overlaps the previous turn; used to wrap a long, straight body part or a body part of increasing circumference

    e. Crinoline, a woven gauze impregnated with Plaster of Paris, is used as a base for casts

    f. Flannel is soft, pliable, and reusable

    g. Muslin is lighter than flannel, strong, and reusable

    h. Elasticized materials apply pressure to an area; can be used as stockings to support and improve venous circulation

2. General information: Binders

    a. Binders wrap specific body parts and are made of flannel, muslin, or elasticized material that fastens with Velcro

    b. Commonly used types are triangular, chest or breast, T, and abdominal binders

    c. A triangular binder, or sling, supports the arm, elbow, or forearm to reduce or prevent swelling

    d. Chest or breast binders provide pressure on the chest or support the breasts

    e. T-binders, either single- or double-tailed, are used to retain pads, dressings, or packs in the perineal area

    f. Abdominal binders, either straight or scultetus (many-tailed), support the abdomen

3. Purpose

    a. To hold dressings in place

    b. To support or immobilize injured body parts

    c. To apply pressure to a wound or body area

    d. To protect an injured body part or area

    e. To prevent additional injury to a body part

    f. To increase client comfort and reduce pain

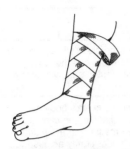 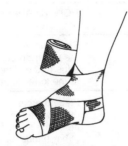 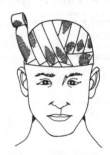

Spiral-reverse: Bandage is anchored first, then reverses direction halfway through each spiral turn; used to accommodate body part of increasing circumference

Figure-eight: Bandage is anchored first below the joint, then alternates ascending and descending turns to form a figure eight; used to turn around joints

Recurrent: Bandage includes a combination of several turns, such as circular, spiral, and spiral-reverse; used to bandage a stump or the scalp

4. Procedure: Applying bandages
   a. Assemble supplies: clean bandages of appropriate size and width, abdominal (ABD) pads or gauze squares to protect bony prominences or prevent two body surfaces from rubbing together, and tape or metal clips to secure the bandage
   b. Wash hands and place the client in a comfortable lying or sitting position that supports the body part
   c. If applying the bandage directly to skin, wash and dry the skin
   d. Pad bony prominences over which the bandage will be placed; use gauze to separate two touching skin surfaces
5. Procedure: Applying binders
   a. Assemble supplies: appropriate binder of correct size and gauze squares to protect bony prominences or prevent two body surfaces from rubbing together
   b. Follow the procedure for applying bandages, but instead of unrolling the bandage, apply the binder (see *Applying binders,* page 136)
6. Documentation
   a. Document bandage or binder application (no need to chart bandages that are used to hold dressings in place)
   b. Note the condition of the skin before application
   c. Record assessment of body part circulation every 1 to 2 hours after application
7. Nursing considerations
   a. Before applying a bandage or binder, inspect the skin for irritation and abrasions and ensure that dressings are clean, dry, and in place
   b. Apply bandages from proximal to distal end to promote venous return

APPLYING BINDERS

TYPE OF BINDER	CLIENT POSITION	HOW TO APPLY
Abdominal	Supine	Place the binder under the client's body, with the upper border at the waist and the lower edge at the gluteal fold; fasten snugly, starting at the lower edge.
Breast	Supine	Place the binder under the client's body with the lower edge at the waist; ask the client to press the sides of the breasts with the palms of her hands; pull the binder tightly across the nipple line; secure with safety pins or Velcro, first at the nipple, then alternately above and below the first fastening.
T	Dorsal recumbent	Place the horizontal band around the client's waist, with vertical tails extending past the buttocks; secure the waistband in front with safety pins; bring single or double center tails between the legs (if single, bring it up over the perineal dressing; if double, bring one tail around each side of the scrotum); fasten tails at the waistband with safety pins placed horizontally.
Triangular	Sitting or supine, with the forearm at an angle (fingers higher than hand, hand higher than wrist, and wrist higher than forearm)	Ask the client to flex the elbow at an 80-degree (or less) angle; place one end of the binder over the unaffected shoulder; extend the bandage over the chest, then under the affected elbow with the point of the triangle under the elbow; bring the lower corner up over the arm to the shoulder of the affected side; tie the two corners with a square knot at shoulder level on the unaffected side.

   c. Bandage the body part in its normal anatomic position, with the joint slightly flexed

   d. Apply bandages smoothly, without wrinkles or creases

   e. Check circulation below the bandaged body part at least every 1 to 2 hours after application

   f. Report coldness, numbness, swelling, pallor, or flushed or cyanotic skin; ask the client to report throbbing, tingling, or pain

   g. Use more than one roller bandage to cover a large area

   h. Reuse a binder until it becomes soiled or wet; a binder can be washed for reuse

Points to Remember

Wound care requires sterile technique because skin integrity is broken.

The surgeon usually performs the first dressing change after surgery.

Wound management involves cleaning the wound, assessing its appearance, and applying sterile dressings.

Key documentation includes a description of the wound and characteristics of any drainage.

Body parts are bandaged in their normal anatomic position.

Circulation of a bandaged body part is assessed at least every 1 to 2 hours after applying the bandage.

Glossary

Closed drainage system — wound drainage system that uses a vacuum to withdraw drainage through tubing into a closed reservoir

Debridement — removal of tissue debris or exudate from a wound

Dehiscence — separation of wound edges

Drain — tube placed in a cavity to permit fluid to escape, usually through suction or gravity

Maceration — skin softening that results from exposure of tissue to moisture

Suture — threadlike material that secures wound edges together

Staple — metal clip or pin that secures wound edges together

Applying Heat and Cold

Learning Objectives

After studying this section, the reader should be able to:

• Describe five methods of applying heat and cold.

• Name the primary effects of heat and cold application.

• Discuss hazards of heat and cold therapy.

• Describe three measures to promote client safety during heat and cold applications.

XI. Applying Heat and Cold

A. Introduction

1. Heat and cold are applied to a client's body to promote tissue repair and healing
   a. The primary effect of heat application is vasodilation, which improves blood flow to the injured body part
   b. Heat application can cause local adverse effects, such as burns or edema, or systemic adverse effects, such as fainting, if enough blood is diverted from the internal organs to cause a drop in blood pressure
   c. The primary effects of cold application are vasoconstriction and slowed metabolism
   d. Cold application alters pain sensation by directly affecting nerve endings and blocking or slowing nerve impulse conduction; cold also reduces muscle spasm by slowing the activity of nerve endings in the muscles
   e. Prolonged exposure to cold causes impaired circulation and tissue damage from oxygen deprivation
2. Clients at risk for burns or tissue injury from heat or cold therapy include:
   a. Elderly clients (because of diminished sensitivity to pain and temperature)
   b. Pediatric clients (because of thin skin layers and a limited ability to verbalize complaints)
   c. Clients with open wounds, stomas, or broken skin (because of limited pain receptors and increased sensitivity of subcutaneous visceral tissues to temperature changes)
   d. Clients with peripheral vascular problems, such as diabetes or arteriosclerosis (because of diminished sensitivity to temperature and pain and further interference with blood flow)
   e. Clients with spinal cord injury or those who are confused or unconscious (because of altered ability to detect sensory or painful stimuli)
3. Heat or cold therapy is administered with dry or moist applications, using clean or sterile technique (see *Comparing dry and moist applications,* page 140)

B. Dry heat application

1. General information
   a. Is applied directly to the body with a hot water bottle, aquathermia pad, or electric heating pad
   b. Is applied indirectly to the body with a heat lamp or heat cradle; less likely to injure tissue because the heat source does not directly touch the skin
   c. May not penetrate into deeper tissue and may increase fluid loss
2. Purpose
   a. To dilate blood vessels in the treated area
   b. To encourage suppuration
   c. To dry weeping or draining wounds

COMPARING DRY AND MOIST APPLICATIONS

Heat and cold applications bring about local and systemic effects to achieve the desired outcome. Heat application raises tissue temperature, causes vasodilation, improves local circulation, increases tissue metabolism, and reduces congestion in deep visceral organs. Cold application stimulates vasoconstriction, inhibits local circulation and tissue metabolism, relieves congestion, slows bacterial activity in infection, reduces body temperature, and acts as a temporary anesthetic.

Heat and cold can be applied in dry or moist forms. The chart below identifies the major advantages and disadvantages of each form.

TYPE OF APPLICATION	ADVANTAGES	DISADVANTAGES
Dry application	• Reduces risk of skin maceration	• Does not penetrate deeply into tissue • Causes increased skin drying
Dry heat	• Is less likely to burn the skin • Permits application at higher temperatures • Can be used for prolonged periods	• Increases body fluid loss through sweating
Dry cold	• Is usually comfortable for the client	• Can cause tissue ischemia with prolonged exposure • Requires a cloth or covering to prevent direct contact with the client's skin
Moist application	• Minimizes skin dryness • Softens wound exudate • Penetrates deeply into tissue • Conforms well to body area being treated	• Can cause skin maceration with prolonged exposure
Moist heat	• Does not result in increased fluid loss from sweating • Is usually comfortable for the client	• Cools rapidly because of evaporation • Creates a greater risk for burns
Moist cold	• Facilitates conduction of cold to penetrate tissues • Suppresses inflammation • Provides local anesthetic effect • Can significantly reduce pain and immobility	• Creates a greater risk for ischemic tissue damage because of deep penetration

    e. To reduce swelling or pain

    f. To increase joint flexibility

    g. To promote healing

3. Procedure: Applying a hot water bottle

    a. Read the physician's order and the nursing care plan for client-specific instructions

    b. Assemble supplies and equipment: hot water bottle, tap water, towel or bottle cover, tape or gauze ties to secure the bottle, and bath blanket (if a large body area will be exposed)

    c. Inspect the client's skin for rash, irritation, or excoriation; thoroughly dry the skin at and near the application site

    d. Drape the client so that only the area to be treated is exposed

    e. Fill the hot water bottle two-thirds full with water at 115° F (46° C); squeeze excess water from the bag and secure the stopper tightly; dry the outside of the bag and cover with a towel or bottle cover

    f. Apply the bottle to the body area, and monitor the site for 5 minutes to avoid burns

    g. Inspect the skin for redness, and ask the client to report pain or discomfort; discontinue therapy if redness or pain occurs

    h. Remove the bottle after the prescribed duration, usually 15 to 20 minutes

4. Procedure: Applying an aquathermia pad

    a. Prepare the client as for a hot water bottle application

    b. Plug in the aquathermia unit to test for proper functioning before taking it to the client's room: check for frayed or exposed wires and cracked plugs to prevent injury

    c. Fill the aquathermia unit two-thirds full with distilled water, and secure the top; regulate the temperature with a key if the unit is not preset

    d. Plug the unit into an outlet, and cover the pad with a bath towel or pillowcase

    e. Continue the procedure as for a hot water bottle application

5. Procedure: Applying a heating pad

    a. Prepare the client as for a hot water bottle application, and test the heating pad as for an aquathermia unit

    b. Cover the heating pad and plug it into an outlet

    c. Set the control at the prescribed temperature

    d. Ensure that the client's skin is dry before applying the pad; tell the client not to change the setting or to lie directly on the pad

    e. Continue the procedure as for a hot water bottle application

6. Procedure: Applying a heat lamp

    a. Prepare the client as for a hot water bottle application, and test the heat lamp as for an aquathermia unit

    b. Plug in the heat lamp

    c. Place the lamp with a 60-watt bulb 18" to 24" (46 to 61 cm) from the area being treated; place the lamp with a larger-watt bulb 24" to 30" (61 to 76 cm) from the area

    d. Do not cover the heat lamp

   e. Continue the procedure as for a hot water bottle application

  7. Procedure: Applying a heat cradle

   a. Prepare the client as for a hot water bottle application, and test the heat cradle as for an aquathermia unit

   b. Fold top bedclothes to the bottom of the bed to make room for the heat cradle

   c. Drape the client so that the area to be treated is exposed

   d. Place the cradle over the area to be treated

   e. Plug in the cradle and cover it and the client with a bath blanket or sheet

   f. Continue the procedure as for a hot water bottle application

  8. Documentation

   a. Record the duration of treatment (start and end times) and the type and site of application

   b. Record the client's skin condition before and after the application

   c. Chart the client's response to the treatment

  9. Nursing considerations

   a. Know that a nurse's primary responsibility when applying heat is to protect a client from injury

   b. Time all heat applications carefully

   c. Notify the physician if the client's skin becomes red or sensitive

   d. Identify a client at risk for injury; the nurse should stay with a client who cannot move or feel pain and should check the client's skin every 5 minutes

   e. Place the call signal within easy reach of the client

C. Moist heat application

  1. General information

   a. Is applied to the body with sterile or unsterile compresses or packs and by soaks or sitz baths

   b. Softens wound exudate, penetrates deeply into tissues, and conforms easily to body parts

   c. Carries increased risk of burns, cools rapidly, and may result in skin maceration

  2. Types

   a. A *compress* is a moist dressing or washcloth applied to a small body area and changed frequently during the designated application time

   b. A *pack* is a moist dressing or towel applied to a large body area

   c. A *soak* is a warm or hot (usually 105° to 110° F [40.5° to 43° C]) solution of tap water, normal saline, or prescribed medication, such as povidone-iodine, in which a body part, such as an arm or leg, is immersed or a sterile or unsterile gauze dressing saturated with solution in which a body part is wrapped

   d. A *sitz bath* is used to soak a client's perineal-rectal area; the client sits immersed from mid-thigh to iliac crest in a special, usually disposable, tub; water temperature ranges from 100° to 115° F (38° to 46° C), depending on the client's age and tolerance

3. Purpose
    a. To relieve pain and enhance client comfort
    b. To promote healing, soften exudate, and hasten suppuration
    c. To clean the wound of tissue debris or exudate
    d. To soothe skin irritation or rash
    e. To apply medication to large skin areas, such as for eczema
    f. To relax muscles
4. Procedure: Applying compresses or packs
    a. Consult the physician's order for the type, duration, and frequency of treatment
    b. Assemble equipment and supplies: basin or sitz bath tub; prescribed solution at correct temperature (if not specified, follow institution policy, usually 105° to 110° F [40.5° to 43° C]); thermometer; forceps; clean towel or washcloth; dressing materials; bath blanket; plastic bag; clean disposable gloves; sterile gloves if indicated; plastic wrap, waterproof pad, and aquathermia pad if applying warm compresses or packs in bed; and tape or tie tapes (Montgomery straps)
    c. Assess the skin for circulatory impairment in the area to be treated; drape a bath blanket as needed to expose only the area to be treated
    d. Place a waterproof pad under the client, and prepare an aquathermia pad
    e. Use sterile technique if the client has an open wound: open sterile supplies and pour warm solution into a sterile container; place gauze in the sterile solution
    f. If using clean technique, place a clean towel or washcloth in warm solution, such as water
    g. Don clean gloves to remove any dressings; discard dressings and gloves in a plastic bag
    h. Don sterile gloves, if necessary; wring out hot compresses with forceps; wring out a warm, clean towel or washcloth by hand
    i. Apply a towel, washcloth, or gauze over the affected area for several seconds; remove material and check the skin for redness; if no redness appears, replace material
    j. Tell the client to notify the nurse if the temperature of the compress or pack is uncomfortable
    k. Apply a plastic wrap or an aquathermia pad over the warm compress or pack; to prevent burns, keep the heating device below 105° F (40.5° C)
    l. Place a towel over the aquathermia pad, and secure it with tape or tie tapes
    m. Maintain treatment for 20 minutes or as ordered
    n. Remove warm applications, dry the client's skin, and apply dressings as ordered, using sterile technique if the client has an open wound
5. Procedure: Soaking a body part
    a. Assemble supplies: sterile or clean container and solution at correct temperature (tap water can be used because it is generally free from pathogens)

    b. Position the solution container so that the client is comfortable and is in proper body alignment

    c. Immerse the body part in the solution for the prescribed time

    d. Add or replace hot solution; try to keep the temperature constant

    e. Continue the soaking for 15 to 20 minutes

    f. End the soaking and dry the body part thoroughly

    g. Dispose of the solution, and clean the equipment

6. Procedure: Giving a sitz bath

    a. Assemble equipment and supplies: sitz bath tub, clean disposable gloves, plastic bag, and bath blanket

    b. Assess the perineal-rectal area; don gloves and remove any dressings; discard dressings and gloves in a plastic bag

    c. Fill a clean bathtub or disposable sitz bath one-third full of water at 100° to 115° F (38° to 46° C); a specially designed sitz tub is preferred to a regular bathtub because the client's legs and feet can be out of the water while the buttocks fit into a deep seat filled with water

    d. Assist the client to and from the bath area; do not leave the client alone if safety is a concern

    e. Place a bath blanket over the client's shoulders and knees during the sitz bath

    f. Have the client sit in the bath for 15 to 30 minutes; add hot water as needed to maintain the prescribed temperature

    g. Help the client to dry thoroughly after the bath

    h. Redress the wound as needed

    i. Tell the client to lie in bed for 30 minutes to permit circulation to return to normal

    j. Dispose of soiled materials, and clean equipment for reuse

7. Documentation

    a. Record the type of moist heat applied, body area treated, and duration of treatment

    b. Chart the appearance of the treated area before and after the procedure

    c. Document the amount and characteristics of any drainage

    d. Record removal and reapplication of any dressings

    e. Note the client's reaction to treatment, including tolerance of the procedure and relief of symptoms, such as pain or itching

8. Nursing considerations

    a. Observe the client for weakness and fatigue; discontinue a bath or soak if the client becomes faint, nauseated, or pallid or develops a rapid pulse

    b. Use a bath thermometer to maintain the prescribed water temperature

    c. Discontinue therapy if the client reports a burning sensation or if the skin reddens

    d. Encourage a client who has had rectal surgery or delivered a baby to take a sitz bath after every bowel movement or as needed for pain relief, unless contraindicated

    e. Tell the client not to touch a wound or scratch affected areas to prevent injury and contamination with pathogens

D. Dry cold application
  1. General information
      a. Dry cold is applied to a small, localized area with an ice bag, ice collar, ice glove, or disposable cold pack
      b. An *ice bag* is made of heavy rubber or plastic and closes tightly; commercially prepared, reusable ice bags are filled with a chemical substance that, once frozen, maintains a cold temperature
      c. An *ice collar* is a narrow, usually disposable, plastic bag used after throat, jaw, or nose surgery
      d. An *ice glove* is a rubber or plastic glove filled with ice chips and tied at the open end; used for small body parts
      e. A *disposable cold pack* contains a chemical that produces cold when the pack is struck, kneaded, or squeezed; commonly used as an alternative to an ice bag, collar, or glove to treat injuries to small body areas, such as an ankle or wrist
  2. Purpose
      a. To reduce acute local inflammation or edema
      b. To decrease or prevent bleeding
      c. To reduce or relieve muscle pain or spasm
      d. To relieve headache caused by vasodilation
  3. Procedure: Applying dry cold
      a. Assemble equipment and supplies as required by the physician's order: ice bag, collar, or glove or cold pack; cloth, towel, or washcloth; bath blanket or pillow; bandage
      b. Fill an ice bag, ice collar, or ice glove one-third to two-thirds full with ice chips; partial filling makes the device lighter and more pliable
      c. Bend the device to remove excess air; insert the stopper securely or tie a knot in the glove's open end
      d. Hold the device upside down to check for leaks
      e. Strike, knead, or squeeze a cold pack to activate its chemicals
      f. Cover the device with a cloth, washcloth, or small towel; use paper tape to hold a washcloth or towel in place
      g. Apply the device and secure it with pillows, an elastic bandage, a roller bandage, or a bath blanket as needed
      h. Inspect the skin after 5 minutes; look for pallor, mottling, cyanosis, or redness
      i. Assess the client's comfort level every 5 to 10 minutes while the device is in place
      j. Remove the application at the designated time, usually after 30 minutes
  4. Documentation
      a. Record the type, site, and duration of application
      b. Document the site's general condition and circulatory status before, during, and after application
      c. Note the client's response to treatment, including tolerance of the procedure and relief of pain, swelling, or bleeding

5. Nursing considerations
    a. Assess the client's skin at least every 10 minutes during the treatment
    b. Palpate peripheral pulses distal to the application site if the skin becomes mottled or cyanotic or the client reports burning or numbness at the site
    c. Prevent sudden chills by exposing only the area to be treated and draping the client with a bath blanket

E. Moist cold application
1. General information
    a. Moist cold applications, which can be sterile or unsterile, include cold compresses or packs and cooling sponge or tub baths using water, water and alcohol, or water and ice
    b. Cold compresses and packs are used to relieve inflammation, prevent edema, and stop bleeding
    c. An ideal sponge bath uses water alone, at a temperature of about 85° to 90° F (29.5° to 32° C)
    d. Although it can rapidly reduce elevated body temperature, alcohol is used sparingly because it dries the skin
    e. Some institutions require a physician's order for application of moist cold; others permit nurses to decide when treatment is necessary
2. Purpose
    a. To reduce marked elevations in body temperature
    b. To relieve local swelling and pain
3. Procedure: Applying cold compresses or packs
    a. Gather equipment: ice, water, gauze or cloth for a compress, ice bag or cooling device
    b. Place water and ice into a clean basin
    c. Immerse gauze or a washcloth, using a size appropriate for the area being treated
    d. Place a waterproof pad on the bed
    e. Wring a compress or pack thoroughly to prevent dripping, and apply it to the affected area
    f. Use an ice bag or commercial cooling device to keep the compress or pack cold
    g. Continue treatment for 20 minutes; repeat every 2 to 3 hours or as ordered by physician
4. Procedure: Giving a sponge bath
    a. Assemble equipment: solution container, solution at appropriate temperature, thermometer, waterproof pad, bath blanket, and gauze, washcloth, or towel
    b. Prepare bath water at a temperature of about 85° to 90° F (29.5° to 32° C)
    c. Protect the bed with a waterproof pad
    d. Drape the client with a bath blanket, exposing only the area to be bathed, to prevent shivering
    e. Apply ice bags as necessary to the head, groin, and axillae

    f. Sponge the client's face and forehead, neck, arms, and legs for 3 to 5 minutes and the back for 10 minutes; cover, but do not dry, each part after it is sponged

    g. Continue bathing the client for 25 to 30 minutes, adding fresh hot water as needed to maintain the desired water temperature

    h. Assess the client's skin color and pulse rate during treatment

    i. Pat the client dry when the bath is completed; assess body temperature 30 minutes later

5. Documentation

    a. Record the type of procedure, the time performed, and the client's response

    b. Document the client's body temperature and skin condition before and after the procedure

6. Nursing considerations

    a. Check the client's pulse rate and skin color during a sponge bath; discontinue therapy if the client reacts poorly (develops shivering chills or complains of numbness or tingling)

    b. Stop any cooling procedure if the client's skin becomes cyanotic or mottled; assess vital signs and check for frostbite

    c. If the client complains of being cold, apply heat to the soles and place a bath blanket over unaffected areas

    d. Use sterile technique when applying cold compresses to an open wound

Points to Remember

Clients at risk for injury from heat or cold applications include pediatric and elderly clients; those with broken skin, open wounds, or stomas; those who are confused or unconscious; those with spinal cord injury; and those with peripheral vascular problems, such as diabetes and arteriosclerosis.

The nurse should consider the client's age, the body part to be treated, and the purpose and type of treatment when determining the safe temperature of the heat or cold application.

The nurse should inspect the skin surface before, during, and after any heat or cold therapy.

The nurse should assess the client every 5 to 10 minutes during the application for unexpected or dangerous reactions.

All applications require careful timing.

Glossary

Aquathermia pad — tubularly constructed pad attached to an electrical source that circulates warm water, providing controlled temperature for heat applications

Compress — wet or dry, cold or warm cloth pad applied to a body part

Mottling — blue-gray to purplish skin blotches caused by peripheral vasoconstriction

Suppuration — formation and discharge of pus

Promoting Oxygenation

Learning Objectives

After studying this section, the reader should be able to:

● Teach a client controlled coughing and deep breathing exercises.

● Identify signs of hypoxia and hypoxemia.

● Describe the procedures for applying a nasal cannula, inserting a nasal catheter, and applying an oxygen mask.

● Review the procedure for suctioning the oropharynx.

● Discuss nursing considerations for tracheostomy care.

● Describe the purpose of closed chest drainage systems.

XII. Promoting Oxygenation

A. **Introduction**
   1. Oxygenation is the process that supplies oxygen to the blood and cells; without adequate oxygen, cells cannot survive
   2. During respiration, oxygen and carbon dioxide are exchanged between the individual and the external environment
   3. The three phases of adequate respiratory function are:
      a. Pulmonary ventilation (inhalation and exhalation of air between the atmosphere and the alveoli of the lungs)
      b. Perfusion (diffusion or movement of oxygen and carbon dioxide between the alveoli and the pulmonary capillaries)
      c. Gas exchange (transport of oxygen and carbon dioxide via the blood to and from the cells)
   4. Inadequate respiratory function results from interference with one or more of these phases and can be caused by:
      a. Airway obstruction
      b. Circulatory malfunction
      c. Inadequate exchange of oxygen and carbon dioxide
      d. Disturbance in the body's acid-base balance
   5. Hypoxemia can result from inadequate respiratory function; the most common signs of hypoxemia are:
      a. Tachycardia
      b. Dyspnea (gasping or irregular respirations)
      c. Restlessness
      d. Flaring nostrils
      e. Cyanosis (blue skin color)
      f. Substernal or intercostal retractions
      g. Increased blood pressure followed by decreased blood pressure
   6. Nursing actions and procedures are directed toward improving and maintaining pulmonary ventilation and preventing hypoxemia
      a. Independent procedures include controlled coughing and deep breathing exercises and incentive spirometry
      b. Interdependent and dependent procedures include postural drainage, oxygen therapy, suctioning, and tracheostomy or chest tube care

B. **Controlled coughing and deep breathing exercises**
   1. General information
      a. Coughing is a natural defense mechanism that protects the lungs and airways from inhaled particles, foreign bodies, and excess secretions
      b. Deep breathing is a means of maximizing normal respiratory volume
      c. The ability to cough and breathe deeply may be diminished in a client with obstructive lung disease, postoperative pain, immobility, or an artificial airway or in one who has received anesthesia or is receiving analgesics or sedatives

      d. Voluntary controlled coughing clears the airways before secretions accumulate; voluntary deep breathing exercises improve ventilation

      e. Deep breathing exercises are taught to those at risk for respiratory problems, such as surgical clients; pursed-lip breathing is taught to clients with alveolar distention to increase effective exhalation and decrease the work of breathing

2. Purpose
      a. To loosen secretions
      b. To promote full lung expansion
      c. To clear airways of pulmonary secretions
      d. To encourage a more effective cough
      e. To improve pulmonary ventilation

3. Procedure: Teaching controlled coughing
      a. Assemble supplies: facial tissues, pillow or folded bath blanket, and stethoscope to assess breath sounds
      b. Help the client to a high Fowler's or upright position in the bed or a chair
      c. Place tissues within easy reach
      d. If the client has an abdominal incision, support the incision either by placing a palm on either side of it or by holding a pillow or folded bath blanket firmly against it
      e. Instruct the client to take several deep breaths and then to inhale deeply, hold it for a second, contract the abdominal muscles, and cough into a tissue
      f. Encourage the client to cough frequently until the airway is cleared or as ordered by the physician

4. Procedure: Teaching deep breathing exercises
      a. Assemble supplies: bath blanket or robe and client's slippers
      b. Help the client to an upright position in the bed or a chair, with both feet on the floor
      c. Place palms around the sides of the client's lower ribs
      d. Instruct the client to inhale slowly and deeply through the nose, expanding the chest and abdominal muscles and concentrating on feeling the abdomen rise
      e. Have the client exhale slowly
      f. Tell the client to repeat this breathing technique, and assess the breathing
      g. Discuss with the client the number and frequency of deep breathing exercises to perform, usually at least five respirations four times a day

5. Procedure: Teaching pursed-lip breathing
      a. Follow the procedure for deep breathing exercises, except for exhalation
      b. Have the client purse lips as if kissing or whistling
      c. Instruct the client to exhale slowly and completely and to avoid puffing out the cheeks; this helps create resistance against air flowing from the lungs and increases pressure within the bronchi, forcing full lung expansion

  d. Discuss with the client the number and frequency of pursed-lip breathing exercises to perform, usually at least five respirations four times a day
6. Documentation
  a. Record the procedure, the time performed, and either duration of treatment or number of coughs or deep breaths
  b. Note the client's response to therapy and ability to perform exercises independently
  c. Chart characteristics of the client's breathing pattern and lung sounds and any signs of dyspnea before and after the procedure
  d. Document the amount and characteristics of any sputum
7. Nursing considerations
  a. Have the client demonstrate the controlled coughing or breathing exercises
  b. Observe the client perform controlled coughing or deep breathing exercises at least once per shift
  c. Reinforce the correct method of controlled coughing or deep breathing if the client is not performing exercises correctly
  d. Auscultate breath sounds before and after coughing or deep breathing exercises

C. Incentive spirometry
1. General information
  a. A spirometer measures the volume of air inhaled (volume spirometer) or the force of air inhaled (flow spirometer) by the client (see *Incentive spirometers*)
  b. The instrument helps the client attain maximal ventilation through slow, deliberate inhalation and exhalation
  c. Incentive spirometry encourages maximal ventilation by establishing alveolar hyperventilation for a time longer than that possible with normal deep breathing, preventing and reversing alveolar collapse produced by such conditions as atelectasis and pneumonitis
  d. Some spirometers are disposable; others are designed for reuse after disinfection
2. Purpose
  a. To promote deep breathing and full expansion of the alveoli
  b. To encourage expectoration of retained secretions
3. Procedure: Teaching incentive spirometry
  a. Assemble equipment and supplies: tissues, volume or flow spirometer, stethoscope, sputum container, and sterile container if specimen must be obtained
  b. Wash hands
  c. Have the client hold a flow spirometer upright; place a volume spirometer on a flat surface within the client's reach
  d. Help the client to an upright position, and place the mouthpiece correctly
  e. Instruct the client to seal his lips tightly around the mouthpiece, take a deep breath, and hold it for 3 seconds

INCENTIVE SPIROMETERS

The illustrations below depict the two major types of incentive spirometer. A *flow spirometer* consists of one or more plastic chambers, each of which contains a movable colored ball that rises on inhalation. In a multi-chambered device, each ball is increasingly weighted so that the ball in the first chamber is lighter than the ball in the next chamber; the heavier the ball, the greater the lung expansion needed to cause the ball to rise.

A *volume spirometer* consists of bellows, a gauge, or a column of lights set at a prescribed volume; raising of the bellows, movement of the gauge, or illumination of the lights indicates how deeply the client is breathing.

Flow spirometer

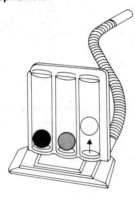

Volume spirometer

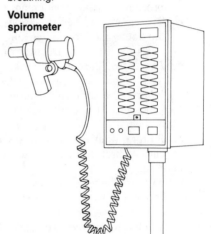

f. If the client is using a flow spirometer, watch the balls rise to note the flow of air; for a volume spirometer, observe the gauge to determine if the client inhales the prescribed volume

g. Remove the mouthpiece and tell the client to exhale slowly and completely

h. Repeat the procedure five times; then ask the client to cough

i. Obtain a sputum specimen, if ordered

j. Clean the mouthpiece with saline solution or cool water; store until the next use

4. Documentation

a. Record the time, type of spirometer used, and duration of treatment or number of inhalations

b. Note the client's response, including lung and breath sounds before and after the procedure, breathing pattern, and any signs of dyspnea

c. Document characteristics of any sputum

5. Nursing considerations

a. Discuss with the client the desired frequency and duration of incentive spirometry

b. Assist until the client can handle the equipment and perform the procedure without help

c. Assess the client's performance of the procedure at least once per shift

D. Postural drainage

1. General information
   a. Postural drainage relies on gravity to drain secretions from various lung segments
   b. A nurse, physical therapist, or respiratory therapist usually performs the procedure, using positioning, percussion, and vibration
   c. The client is placed in various positions so that congested lung segments are above the airways, enabling secretions to drain by gravity; lower lobes require more frequent drainage
   d. *Percussion,* the forceful striking of the skin with cupped hands, is used to dislodge secretions for expectoration
   e. *Vibration,* a series of vigorous contractions and relaxations produced by hands placed flat against the chest wall, loosens secretions from the bronchial tree to the trachea
   f. Postural drainage is especially effective in a client with cystic fibrosis, chronic bronchitis, emphysema, asthma, pneumonia, or lung infiltration

2. Purpose
   a. To loosen lung secretions
   b. To clear airways of pulmonary secretions
   c. To encourage more effective coughing
   d. To improve pulmonary ventilation

3. Procedure: Performing postural drainage
   a. Place the client in a position appropriate for draining the affected lung segment (see *Positioning a client for postural drainage,* pages 155 and 156)
   b. Help the client maintain the appropriate position for 10 to 15 minutes to ensure adequate drainage of the lung segment
   c. Cover the area to be percussed with a towel or gown, and percuss for 1 to 2 minutes over the lung segment by alternately tapping the cupped hands over the area
   d. Vibrate by placing flattened hands one over the other or side by side against the affected chest area
   e. Have the client inhale and then exhale through pursed lips
   f. Alternately contract and relax fingers placed against the chest wall for 8 to 10 seconds while the client exhales
   g. Repeat the procedure for 2 to 5 minutes, depending on the client's tolerance and amount of secretions expelled

4. Documentation
   a. Record the procedure, time performed, duration of treatment, and positions used
   b. Note the client's response, including lung and breath sounds before and after the procedure, breathing pattern, or signs of dyspnea

POSITIONING A CLIENT FOR POSTURAL DRAINAGE

To drain the *posterior basal segments of the lower lobes,* elevate the foot of the table 18″ (46 cm) or 30 degrees, or change the elevation of the foot of the bed similarly. Position the client on his abdomen with head lowered. Place pillows as shown. Percuss the lower ribs on both sides of the spine.

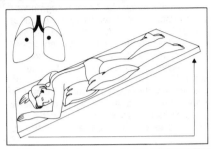

To drain the *lateral basal segments of the lower lobes,* elevate the foot of the table or bed 18″ or 30 degrees. Position the client on his abdomen with head lowered and upper leg flexed over a pillow for support. Have him rotate a quarter turn upward. Percuss the lower ribs on the uppermost portion of the lateral chest wall.

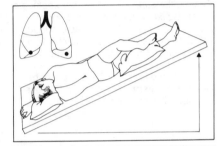

To drain the *anterior basal segments of the lower lobes,* elevate the foot of the table or bed 18″ or 30 degrees. Position the client on his side with his head lowered. Place pillows as shown. Percuss with a slightly cupped hand over the lower ribs just beneath the axilla. *Note:* If an acutely ill client experiences breathing difficulty in this position, adjust the angle of the table or bed to one he can tolerate. Then begin percussion.

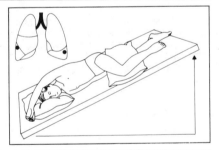

To drain the *superior segments of the lower lobes,* keep the table or bed flat. Position the client on his abdomen, and place two pillows under his hips. Percuss on both sides of the spine at the lower tip of the scapulae.

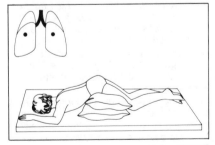

(continued)

POSITIONING A CLIENT FOR POSTURAL DRAINAGE *(continued)*

To drain the *medial and lateral segments of the right middle lobe,* elevate the foot of the table or bed 14" (36 cm) or 15 degrees. Position the client on his left side with his head lowered and knees flexed. Then have him rotate a quarter turn backward. Place a pillow beneath him. Percuss with the hand moderately cupped over the right nipple. For a female client, cup the hand so its heel is under the armpit and fingers extend forward beneath the breast.

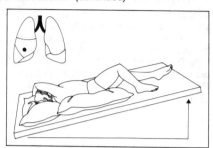

To drain the *superior and inferior segments of the lingular portion of the left upper lobe,* elevate the foot of the table or bed 14" or 15 degrees. Position the client on his right side with his head lowered and knees flexed. Then have him rotate a quarter turn backward. Place a pillow behind him from shoulders to hips. Percuss as above, but on the left side.

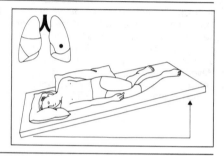

To drain the *anterior segments of the upper lobes,* keep the table or bed flat. Have the client lie on his back with a pillow folded under his knees. Then have him rotate slightly away from the side being drained. Percuss between the clavicle and nipple.

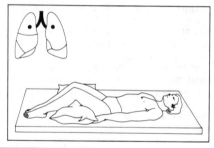

To drain the *apical segment of the right upper lobe and the apical subsegment of the left upper lobe,* have the client sit on a flat table or bed. Standing behind the client and holding a pillow, have him lean back on the pillow at a 30-degree angle. Percuss between the clavicle and the top of each scapula.

To drain the *posterior segment of the right upper lobe and the posterior subsegment of the left upper lobe,* have the client sit and lean over a folded pillow at a 30-degree angle. Standing behind him, percuss and clap the upper back on each side.

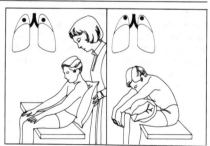

    c. Chart the amount and characteristics of sputum and, if applicable, collection of sputum specimen and the time it was sent to the laboratory

5. Nursing considerations
    a. Schedule postural drainage at least 30 minutes to 1 hour after the client eats to prevent nausea, vomiting, and possible aspiration
    b. Encourage the client to drink 8 to 12 8-oz glasses (2 to 3 liters) of fluids daily to liquefy pulmonary secretions
    c. Avoid percussing over the spine, liver, kidneys, or spleen to prevent injury
    d. Help the client clean and freshen the mouth with mouthwash after the procedure
    e. Auscultate the client's lungs before and after the procedure, and compare with baseline data

E. Oxygen therapy

1. General information
    a. Oxygen therapy refers to the administration of supplemental oxygen by a device, such as a nasal cannula, nasal catheter, or mask
    b. The procedure is indicated after surgery or for any condition that causes hypoxia, such as pneumonia, congestive heart failure, lung tumors, or degenerative lung diseases
    c. A dependent nursing function, oxygen therapy requires a physician's order specifying administration method, amount of oxygen to be given, and duration of treatment
    d. Special storage facilities, flow control devices, humidifying devices, and oxygen delivery equipment are required

2. Hypoxia and hypoxemia
    a. *Hypoxia* is an inadequate amount of oxygen to meet the metabolic needs of tissues and cells; *hypoxemia* is a deficiency of oxygen in arterial blood
    b. Signs of hypoxia include hypotension, arrhythmias, tachypnea, dyspnea, headache, and disorientation; arterial blood gas (ABG) studies, especially of partial pressures of oxygen and carbon dioxide, are needed for confirmation
    c. Signs of hypoxemia, in order of occurrence, are increased rapid pulse, rapid shallow respirations, dyspnea, increased restlessness or light-headedness, flaring of nostrils, substernal or intercostal retractions, and cyanosis

3. Oxygen
    a. Oxygen—a colorless, tasteless, odorless gas—is a safety hazard if exposed to intense heat, combustible materials, sparks, or fire
    b. Because oxygen is a dry gas, it dehydrates both tissues and secretions; it is humidified by adding water through a bubbler or nebulizer
    c. Oxygen is available at bedside through piped-in (or wall) and portable (in a cylinder) units

   d. Piped-in oxygen is stored in a large central reservoir under enough
      pressure to flood a system of pipes and outlets at bedside units or other
      locations, such as operating rooms
   e. Portable oxygen is stored in small or large green cylinders under high
      pressure and labeled "oxygen"; large cylinders can be heavy and difficult
      to handle
   f. Oxygen flow is controlled by a flow meter, an instrument that regulates
      the amount of oxygen (in liters/minute) released from a source
   g. Oxygen is delivered through a tube attached to a low-flow device
      (delivers oxygen in concentrations below 40%, depending on the rate and
      depth of client breathing) or a high-flow device (delivers controlled,
      precise amounts of oxygen in higher concentrations)
   h. The type of oxygen delivery device ordered by the physician is
      determined by the client's condition and needs (see *Comparing oxygen
      delivery devices,* pages 160 to 163)
4. Purpose
   a. To provide oxygen to a client with hypoxia or hypoxemia
   b. To provide oxygen to a client at risk for hypoxia or hypoxemia (for
      example, to a woman in labor with a fetus at risk for hypoxia)
5. Procedure: Administering oxygen with a nasal cannula
   a. Assess the client for signs and symptoms of hypoxia; ensure a patent
      airway and remove airway secretions if necessary; review the client's
      most recent ABG results
   b. Consult the physician's order for oxygen delivery method, flow rate, and
      duration of therapy; notify the institution's respiratory therapy
      department, if one exists
   c. Assemble required oxygen delivery equipment: nasal cannula, oxygen
      tubing, oxygen source, distilled water for humidification, flow meter
   d. Wash hands; then add sterile distilled water to the indicated level on the
      humidification bottle, or use a prefilled, disposable bag or bottle
   e. Attach a nasal cannula to the humidified oxygen source, using connective
      tubing as necessary
   f. Adjust the oxygen flow rate to the prescribed amount; if the physician's
      order does not specify a rate, set at 2 liters/minute and then ask the
      physician for a specific rate
   g. Ensure that oxygen is flowing from the cannula outlets and that water in
      the humidifying device is bubbling
   h. Place the cannula tips or nasal prongs into the client's nostrils
   i. Adjust the tubing around the client's ears, and use a plastic slide to
      secure the tubing under the chin or place an elastic band around the
      client's head above the ears
   j. Provide sufficient slack in the tubing, and secure it to the client's gown
   k. Recheck and adjust oxygen flow as necessary to maintain the prescribed
      rate
6. Procedure: Administering oxygen with a nasal catheter
   a. Follow the first four steps for using a nasal cannula

b. Place the client in semi-Fowler's position

c. Cut a 4″ to 5″ (10 to 13 cm) strip of tape, and slit one end vertically about 2″ (5 cm)

d. Measure and mark the catheter from the tip of the client's nose to the earlobe

e. Connect the catheter to the oxygen source with tubing

f. Adjust the flow rate to the prescribed amount; if not specified, set at 2 liters/minute and obtain the physician's order as soon as possible

g. Lubricate the tip of the nasal catheter with water-soluble lubricant

h. Gently insert the catheter into a nostril, guiding it medially along the floor of the nasal cavity until the marked point is at the nostril edge; oxygen flow during insertion should prevent the catheter from becoming plugged with secretions

i. Inspect the oral cavity, using a flashlight and tongue blade (the catheter tip should be seen at the side of the uvula)

j. Place the tape's uncut edge on the client's nose, and wrap the split end around the catheter to keep it in place; secure the tubing to the client's gown or bedding with a safety pin

7. Procedure: Administering oxygen with a mask

a. Follow the first four steps for using a nasal cannula

b. Place the client in a semi-Fowler's or high Fowler's position

c. For a simple mask, set oxygen flow to the prescribed amount, usually 6 to 10 liters/minute

d. As the client exhales, position the mask from the nose downward; fasten the elastic band over the client's ears and tighten so that the mask fits snugly

e. Check for leaks around the mask's edges

f. For a Venturi mask, adjust the control device to the prescribed oxygen percentage, and look for visible mist coming from the mask before placing it on the client's face

g. For a partial rebreathing or nonrebreathing mask, open the oxygen flow to 8 to 10 liters/minute; after placing the mask on the client's face, pull it back and slip the thumb over the reservoir bag outlet and allow the bag to fill completely; remove the thumb and adjust the mask as needed

8. Documentation

a. Record the oxygen administration method, the flow rate, and the time therapy began

b. Note the client's response to therapy and any change in his condition

c. Document any unexpected or undesirable effects, such as excoriation around the nose or mouth

9. Nursing considerations

a. Know that administering oxygen (a medication) is a dependent nursing function; the physician's order must indicate the administration method, the amount of oxygen to be given (in liters/minute or the percentage of oxygen concentration), and the duration or frequency of therapy

(Text continues on page 162.)

COMPARING OXYGEN DELIVERY DEVICES

OXYGEN DEVICE

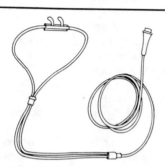

Nasal cannula (flexible plastic tube with two hollow prongs inserted into the nose)

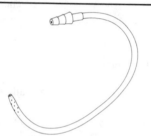

Nasal catheter (flexible plastic tube inserted through the nose into the pharynx)

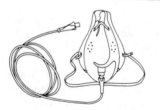

Simple mask (small mask placed over the nose and mouth and held securely in place)

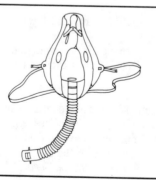

Venturi mask (mask that delivers high concentrations of controlled flow by changing the size of the openings in the device)

ADVANTAGES	DISADVANTAGES
• Simple to attach • Does not interfere with eating or talking • Exerts minimal pressure against skin and mucous membranes • Inexpensive • Disposable • Permits low-flow oxygen therapy	• Cannot deliver oxygen concentrations above 40% • Cannot be used in a client with complete nasal obstruction • Can cause headaches or dry mucous membranes if the flow rate exceeds 6 liters/minute • Can be easily dislodged • Requires client to be alert and cooperative to keep cannula in place
• Permits client to move freely • Does not interfere with eating or talking • Permits low-flow oxygen therapy • Can be set to deliver flow rates of 6 to 10 liters/minute • Delivers 44% to 68% concentration, depending on the client's rate and depth of breathing • Inexpensive • Disposable	• Dries and irritates mucous membranes • Can misdirect oxygen into the stomach • Kinks easily • Must be moved to alternate nostril every 8 hours because the tube irritates mucous membranes • May become clogged with secretions
• Permits low-flow therapy • Delivers a rate of 6 to 10 liters/minute • Delivers 44% to 68% concentration, depending on the client's rate and depth of breathing	• Uncomfortable because of required close fit over the nose and mouth • Can cause excoriation of skin because of close fit and accumulation of moisture from condensation • Interferes with drinking, eating, and talking • Impractical for long-term therapy
• Delivers 2 to 10 liters/minute • Delivers precise 24% to 44% concentration regardless of client's respiratory pattern because same amount of room air always enters the opening • Permits—but does not require—humidification • Permits high-flow oxygen therapy	• Uncomfortable because of required close fit over the nose and mouth • Causes excoriation of skin from continuous pressure against the face and moisture buildup • Interferes with eating, drinking, and talking

(continued)

COMPARING OXYGEN DELIVERY DEVICES *(continued)*

OXYGEN DEVICE

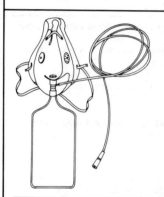

Partial rebreathing mask (similar to the simple mask with a reservoir bag attached to increase potential concentration)

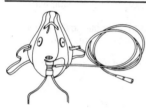

Nonrebreathing mask (mask with a stop-gap valve between the bag and mask that prevents oxygen from mixing with room air)

---

  b. Administer oxygen in emergencies without a physician's order, following institution guidelines for volume and flow rate; obtain a physician's order for oxygen as soon as possible thereafter

  c. Use caution when administering oxygen to a client with chronic lung disease; high oxygen levels can disrupt the breathing stimulus and lead to respiratory arrest

  d. Check the client for signs of hypoxia at least every 2 hours

  e. Assess the oxygen device, the fluid level in the humidification bag or bottle, the flow rate, and the client's nose, nostrils, and surrounding skin for breakdown at least every 4 hours

  f. Adjust oxygen flow to maintain the prescribed rate and fill the humidification bottle or bag as needed (in some institutions, respiratory therapy personnel change the prefilled, disposable humidification bag or bottle at regular intervals or as needed; humidification of oxygen must be maintained to prevent drying of mucous membranes)

  g. Use a water-soluble lubricant for red, irritated skin and mucous membranes; never use petrolatum, which holds moisture against the skin and prevents it from drying

  h. Move the nasal catheter to the client's opposite nostril every 8 hours because the catheter tip irritates mucous membranes

ADVANTAGES	DISADVANTAGES
● Conserves and permits rebreathing of first one-third of exhaled air, which has a high oxygen concentration ● Permits low-flow oxygen therapy ● Delivers up to 10 liters/minute ● Delivers up to 90% concentration ● Permits inhalation of room air through holes in the mask if oxygen source fails	● Causes excoriation of skin ● Uncomfortable because of required close fit over the nose and mouth ● Interferes with eating, drinking, and talking ● Bag may twist or kink ● Impractical for long-term therapy
● Provides highest possible oxygen concentration (up to 95%) ● Delivers 6 to 15 liters/minute ● Can be used to administer an anesthetic ● Permits low-flow oxygen therapy	● Causes excoriation of skin ● Interferes with eating, drinking, and talking ● Impractical for long-term therapy

      i. Check mask size to ensure a snug fit, which prevents oxygen from escaping around the eyes and mouth

      j. Remove the mask briefly every 2 to 4 hours, and wash and dry the skin carefully to prevent excoriation

      k. Raise the mask slightly above the client's face during eating or drinking

      l. At least once per shift (or more frequently, if the client's condition warrants), check ports on a Venturi mask for obstruction (such as from bed linens or the client's gown) to prevent interference with delivery of the correct percentage of oxygen

      m. Follow oxygen safety precautions (see *Safety precautions for using oxygen,* page 164)

F. Suctioning

    1. General information

      a. Suctioning is the aspiration of secretions through a rubber or polyethylene catheter attached to a suction machine or wall suction outlet

      b. Secretions are removed from the upper respiratory tract (oropharyngeal or nasopharyngeal suctioning)

SAFETY PRECAUTIONS FOR USING OXYGEN

● Place "No Smoking" and "Oxygen In Use" signs at the unit where oxygen is being used and on the room door.
● Remove cigarettes, matches, and lighters from the room.
● Disconnect ungrounded electrical equipment.
● Make sure all electrical monitoring equipment is properly grounded.
● Remove all volatile materials, except solutions and equipment to be used during therapy.
● Locate fire extinguishers.
● If using portable oxygen, keep cylinders in a device that prevents them from being knocked over.
● Regard oxygen as a medication that requires a physician's order for administration

---

    c. The catheter, with a port at the distal end, is attached to a suction device and inserted into the pharynx or other part of the airway; suction is applied by placing the thumb over the port

    d. Sterile technique prevents pathogens from entering the pharynx, where they can multiply and invade the trachea and bronchi

    e. The procedure is indicated for a client who cannot cough or swallow or who has accumulated secretions, as evidenced by light bubbling or rattling breath sounds

    f. Suctioning can dry mucous membranes, cause trauma, or (if improperly performed) introduce pathogens into the normally sterile airways, making a client more susceptible to infection

2. Purpose
    a. To remove secretions obstructing the airway
    b. To facilitate respirations
    c. To obtain a specimen for diagnostic purposes
    d. To remove accumulated secretions that can cause infection
    e. To stimulate coughing and deep breathing

3. Procedure: Suctioning the upper respiratory tract
    a. Assess the client's need for suctioning by observing for a decreased or absent cough reflex, impaired pulmonary function, or thick, tenacious mucus; a weak, debilitated, semicomatose, or comatose client is especially vulnerable to accumulated secretions
    b. Assemble equipment and supplies: portable suction machine, tubing, and collection container for wall suction; sterile suction set, including sterile disposable gloves; cup or container for sterile water or normal saline solution; suction catheter, either open-tipped (openings at end and along sides) or whistle-tipped (slanted opening at tip); sterile water or normal saline solution to lubricate and flush catheter; Y connector (if the catheter does not have a thumb port); plastic bag for waste disposal; towel or waterproof pad; and sputum trap if a specimen must be collected

SETTINGS FOR SUCTION GAUGES

Age-group	Wall unit settings	Portable unit settings
Adults	120 to 150 mm Hg	7 to 15 mm Hg
Children	80 to 120 mm Hg	5 to 10 mm Hg
Infants	0 to 100 mm Hg	5 to 10 mm Hg

   c. Place a conscious client with a functional gag reflex in a semi-Fowler's position, with the head turned to one side for oral suctioning or the neck hyperextended for nasal suctioning; place an unconscious client in a sidelying position facing the nurse and extend neck for nasal suctioning

   d. Instruct the client to cough and breathe slowly before suctioning to minimize hypoxia; if the client cannot do so, manually hyperventilate, using a hand-held resuscitation bag

   e. Lay a towel or pad over a pillow on the client's chest to avoid soiling the client

   f. Wash hands; then open the catheter package, leaving the protective covering over the catheter; pour sterile saline solution into the container

   g. Turn on the suction, and adjust the pressure on the suction gauge to the appropriate setting (see *Settings for suction gauges*)

   h. Don gloves (if only one sterile glove is in the package, use a clean glove on one hand to control the on-off button, suction gauge, and suction port)

   i. Connect the catheter to the tubing, grasping the catheter end with the sterile glove and suction tubing with the clean glove

   j. Lubricate the tip and inside of the catheter by dipping it into sterile saline solution and applying suction

   k. Insert the catheter through the client's mouth or nostril without applying suction; never force insertion

   l. Advance the catheter until it reaches the pool of mucus

   m. Begin suctioning by placing a thumb over the suction port or Y connector while withdrawing the catheter with a rotating motion; do not suction for more than 5 to 10 seconds at a time; withdraw the catheter slightly if the client coughs

   n. Allow the client to breathe normally between periods of suctioning; administer oxygen if needed

   o. Flush the catheter after each removal by aspirating saline solution

   p. Continue suctioning until the airway is free of secretions, waiting 1 to 2 minutes before suctioning again to allow the client to breathe and replace air removed during the procedure

   q. Turn off the suction machine; turn a glove over the used catheter and discard it in a lined waste container; wash hands

4. Documentation
    a. Record the procedure, the time performed, and the number of times the client was suctioned
    b. Document the amount, consistency, color, and odor of secretions
    c. Record signs indicating the client's need for suctioning, response to treatment, and respiratory status after the procedure, including changes in breath sounds
5. Nursing considerations
    a. Deeper suctioning of the trachea or bronchi requires considerable skill and is usually performed only by a nurse given special instruction and supervision
    b. The pharyngeal cavity is not suctioned in a client who has had nasopharyngeal surgery or tonsillectomy because of possible trauma to the incision or dislodging of clots, which may cause hemorrhage
    c. Check the client's status before and after suctioning
    d. Use the appropriate catheter size: adults, #12 to #18 French; children, #8 to #10 French; infants, #5 to #8 French
    e. Use sterile technique to prevent introduction of pathogens into the client's airway
    f. If suctioning equipment is not functioning, check that connections for the catheter, suction equipment, and collection bottle plug are secure and tight and that the catheter or tubing is not kinked
    g. To ease catheter insertion into the nostril, insert the catheter on a slight downward slant, and ask the client to take slow deep breaths through his mouth
    h. To reduce trauma, alternate suctioning between left and right nostrils in a client with no history of nasal problems
    i. For oropharyngeal suctioning, depress the client's tongue with a tongue blade to improve sight lines to the back of the throat and to prevent the client from biting on the catheter
    j. After suctioning is completed, keep a sterile catheter at the bedside for the next suctioning or in case of emergency
    k. Empty the suction bottle at the end of each shift or more often if secretions reach the fluid level line on the bottle; wear clean, disposable gloves when emptying the bottle

G. Tracheostomy care
1. General information
    a. A *tracheostomy* is a small opening made in the trachea just below the first or second tracheal cartilage to provide a clear passageway for air
    b. The surgery, called a *tracheotomy,* is performed as an emergency measure because of acute airway obstruction, such as occurs in croup, or because of injury to the airway; a tracheotomy is sometimes performed to create a permanent artificial airway when an alternate airway is needed, such as in laryngeal cancer

    c. The client with a tracheostomy has an increased susceptibility to respiratory infections because the normal protective mechanisms of warming, filtering, and moisturizing the air are bypassed, and the client cannot cough effectively

    d. A tracheostomy renders the client unable to speak or call for assistance, causing emotional stress for the client and family members

    e. The client breathes through a tracheostomy tube (a curved single- or double-lumen tube inserted into the tracheostomy and extending into the trachea); the outer cannula is held in place by ties around the neck; the inner cannula is locked into the outer cannula

    f. The procedure may require use of a tracheostomy cuff (a rubber, balloonlike appliance placed around the lower two-thirds of the outer cannula); after the tube is inserted, the cuff is inflated to prevent accidental removal or air leaks, if positive pressure devices are used

    g. Tracheostomy care requires use of sterile technique

2. Purpose

    a. To maintain a patent airway

    b. To prevent infection

    c. To promote cleanliness and avoid skin breakdown around the tracheostomy

    d. To decrease the work of breathing

3. Procedure: Suctioning a tracheostomy tube and cleaning the inner cannula

    a. Assemble supplies and equipment: tracheal cleaning tray if available (includes sterile basins, pipe cleaners, brush, 4″ × 4″ gauze pads, precut dressings), suction catheter package, sterile normal saline solution, hydrogen peroxide, clean tracheal ties, complete tracheal tie set for emergency use, interchangeable inner cannula of the same size, sterile gloves, and soft washcloth and towel

    b. Wash hands

    c. Follow the procedure for oropharyngeal suctioning, except insert the catheter through the tracheostomy tube until it meets resistance; pull back ½″ (1 cm) and begin suctioning; if necessary, instill a prescribed amount (usually 3 to 5 ml) of sterile normal saline into the tube to help liquefy secretions before suctioning

    d. Open the tracheostomy tray, and pour hydrogen peroxide and saline solution into separate sterile basins

    e. Put on sterile gloves and unlock the inner cannula by turning it to the left about 90 degrees

    f. Hold the outer cannula in place with the left thumb and forefinger; then gently pull the inner cannula slightly up and out

    g. Place the inner cannula in the sterile container of hydrogen peroxide

    h. Clean the inside and outside of the cannula with pipe cleaners or a brush moistened with hydrogen peroxide; rinse with sterile water or saline solution; dry with a sterile gauze pad

    i. Replace by grasping the cannula's outer flange with the left hand while inserting the inner cannula

      j. Lock the inner cannula by turning it to the right

      k. Wash, rinse, and dry the client's neck with a soft washcloth and towel

      l. Clean around the incision site with applicator sticks soaked in normal saline solution or hydrogen peroxide, and apply antibiotic ointment if ordered

      m. Place a precut sterile dressing on the skin around the outer cannula

      n. Cut ties to the correct length, or use precut ties; fold the ends of the ties, and cut a slit starting at the folded edge

      o. Have an assistant hold the outer cannula in place; then cut, remove, and discard the old ties

      p. Pass the slit end of the ties through the flange loop of the tracheostomy tube about 2″ to 3″ (5 to 8 cm); thread the other end of the tie all the way through the slit, pulling it firmly into place

      q. Repeat the procedure on the second flange with the second tie; bring the ties around the client's neck

      r. Tie a square knot to one side of the neck

4. Procedure: Deflating and inflating a tracheal cuff

      a. Check the physician's order (high-volume, low-pressure cuffs are not usually deflated)

      b. Gather equipment: suctioning equipment, 10-ml syringe

      c. Suction the tracheostomy tube before deflating the cuff

      d. Attach a 10-ml syringe to the distal end of the cuff, making sure that the seal is tight

      e. Slowly withdraw about 5 ml of air (the amount is determined by the type of cuff)

      f. Keep the syringe attached; immediately reinflate the cuff if the client's respirations become labored

      g. Suction the tube again before reinflating the cuff

      h. Inject the prescribed amount of air to create a leak-free system; check for leaks by holding a stethoscope over the trachea; a hissing sound indicates correct inflation

      i. Remove the syringe and insert a one-way valve to prevent air leaks

5. Documentation

      a. Document the type and frequency of tracheostomy care

      b. Chart the amount and characteristics of suctioned secretions

      c. Note the client's response to the procedure

      d. Record in the nurses' notes client and family teaching about tracheostomy care in preparation for home care, if appropriate

6. Nursing considerations

      a. Tape an obturator of appropriate size to the head of the client's bed; use it to reinsert an outer cannula that accidentally becomes dislodged

      b. Perform tracheostomy care under sterile conditions; discourage the client from touching the tracheostomy tube

      c. Unless contraindicated, remove the inner cannula every 8 hours for cleaning

d. Check institution policy for alternate methods of applying tracheostomy ties, including use of commercial products that have Velcro or similar fastening devices

e. Check the size of the airway and the tracheostomy tube to determine the volume of air required to inflate the cuff properly

f. Deflate a cuffed tracheostomy tube every 8 hours or as ordered; if a tracheostomy cuff has two balloons, alternately inflate them every hour

g. Never cut gauze near the tracheostomy; threads could enter the airway and cause irritation and infection

h. Send reusable equipment to the supply department for disinfection or sterilization

H. Chest tube care

1. General information

   a. A closed chest drainage system uses chest tubes to remove air or fluid from the pleural cavity, with or without suction; an open drainage system allows air to be sucked into the chest cavity and collapses the lungs

   b. Chest tubes are made of pliable plastic or rubber and are inserted during any surgical procedure in which the chest is opened or during emergency treatment of injuries or diseases that cause pleural leaks

   c. The pressure in the pleural cavity is normally lower than that of the atmosphere (negative pressure), causing air to rush into the chest when an injury, such as a stab wound, occurs; any drainage system connected to the chest must be sealed against air and fluids; if air or fluids enter the pleural space, the lungs collapse (pneumothorax)

   d. When the chest is opened, a vacuum is needed to reestablish negative pressure

   e. Water-sealed chest drainage systems use water as a seal to keep air from being drawn into the pleural space; these systems use one bottle (that collects drainage and maintains a water seal), two bottles (one collects drainage and one maintains a water seal), or three bottles (the third bottle is attached to the suction system)

   f. Disposable pleural drainage systems are also available

2. Purpose

   a. To maintain an airtight system until the client's lungs reexpand and air or fluid is removed from the pleural space

   b. To maintain patency of chest tubes

   c. To maintain a water-sealed system

   d. To promote adequate gaseous exchange until normal respiratory function returns

3. Procedure: Maintaining a chest tube

   a. Assess the client's respiratory status; report rapid, shallow breathing, chest pressure, hemorrhage, pallor, or cyanosis

   b. Keep rubber-tipped hemostats at the bedside; if ordered or in an emergency, clamp the chest tube near the insertion site (chest tube or tubing is not usually pinched or clamped for more than 1 minute)

    c. Monitor the tubes for air leaks; if a leak develops, clamp the tube briefly and notify the physician

    d. If the chest tube becomes dislodged, apply pressure over the area with the hand, a sheet, or other nearby material; immediately alert the physician; sterile petroleum gauze can prevent air leaks

    e. Keep suction bottles or a disposable system below the level of the bed; maintain the water level in a water-seal bottle

    f. Milk the chest tube every hour if ordered (pinch the tubing close to the chest with one hand and milk the tube with the other hand; continue this procedure down the tube, milking away from the client into a drainage container)

    g. Assess functioning of the system by checking drainage and looking for bubbling in the water-seal chamber (indicates entry of air)

    h. If a chest drainage bottle or bag becomes full, change it under negative pressure conditions using sterile technique (a physician's order is required for this procedure); clamp the tube near the chest wall, and change the bottle or bag during inhalation

4. Documentation

    a. Record the amount and color of drainage, and note whether clots are present

    b. Document malfunctioning of the system and measures taken to correct the problem

    c. Note the client's respiratory rate and rhythm and the presence and character of breath sounds

    d. Chart frequency of tube milking

5. Nursing considerations

    a. Keep the drainage system below chest level so that fluid in the container is not drawn into the pleural space by gravity

    b. Change the client's position every 2 hours to encourage drainage of secretions

    c. Teach the client to perform controlled coughing and deep breathing exercises every 2 hours

    d. Encourage increased fluid intake to liquefy secretions

    e. Inspect the dressing around the insertion site for drainage and signs of infection

    f. Expect bubbling in the water-seal chamber if the client has pneumothorax; otherwise, bubbling may indicate a crack in the unit or a leak in the tubing between the pleural cavity and the unit

Points to Remember

Nursing procedures for a client with a respiratory problem are directed toward improving pulmonary ventilation and preventing pulmonary complications.

The nurse should administer oxygen carefully to a client with chronic lung disease because increased oxygen levels can depress respirations.

Safety precautions are imperative during oxygen therapy.

Clinical signs of hypoxia include hypotension, arrhythmias, tachypnea, dyspnea, headache, and disorientation.

Airway suctioning and tracheostomy care require sterile technique.

Glossary

Atelectasis — abnormal respiratory condition in which lung tissue collapses, interfering with gas exchange

Cannula — tube inserted to remove air or secretions from the body

Cyanosis — dusky, gray, or blue color of skin and mucous membranes

Hypoxia — insufficient oxygen supply to cells and tissues

Hypoxemia — lack of oxygen in arterial blood

Obturator — plug with olive-shaped end that fits inside a tracheostomy cannula, preventing tissue damage when the tube is placed in the tracheostomy

Index

i refers to an illustration; t refers to a table.

Sterile technique, 31t
in catheterization, 63
in heat and cold therapy, 139
in I.V. therapy, 109, 114
with open skin lesions, 102, 103
in parenteral medication administration, 95
in suctioning, 164, 166
in tracheostomy care, 167
in wound care, 32, 122, 128, 132, 144, 148
Stridor, 20
Suctioning, 150, 163-166
Suppository, administration of, 105-106
Surgical asepsis. *See* Asepsis.
Suture removal, 129-131
Syringes, specifications of, 95t

T

Tachycardia, 16
Tachypnea, 19t
Temperature, assessment of
axillary, 15
oral, 13-14
rectal, 14-15
Thermometers, 12, 13t, 14, 15
Tracheostomy care, 166-169
Tracheotomy, 166
Transfusion reactions, 118, 119
Trash, disposal of, 29
Trauma, prevention of, 66
Tube
chest, 169-170
Dubbhoff, 74t
enteral, 80-81
Ewald, 74t
Levin, 74t
nasogastric, 73, 74t, 75, 76t, 77-79
rectal, 73, 83-84, 85
Salem sump, 74t
tracheostomy, 168, 169
Tube feedings. *See* Enteral tube feedings.
Typing and crossmatching, 117

UV

Universal body fluid precautions, 27
Urination. *See* Elimination.

Urine specimen collection, 62-63
from indwelling catheter, 66-67
Urinometer, 71
Venipuncture sites, 111, 112i
Venturi mask, 159, 160i, 163
Vibration (technique for postural drainage), 154
Vital signs, assessment of, 12-24
Volume control set, 115, 116

WXYZ

Walking belt, 51, 58
Wound care
bandage application, 133-136
binder application, 133-136
cleaning, 125i
draining, 124-126, 127, 128i
dressing, 122-124, 128-129
irrigating, 132, 133i
staple removal, 129-131
suture removal, 129-131

i refers to an illustration; t refers to a table.

Notes